D0322852

Health Policy and Ethics

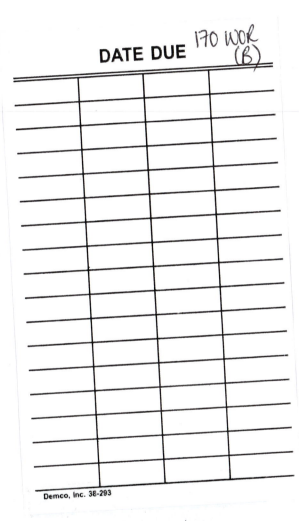

DATE DUE 170 WOR (B)

Demco, Inc. 38-293

Health Policy and Ethics

A Critical Examination of Values from a Global Perspective

ROGER WORTHINGTON PhD

Assistant (Adjunct) Professor of Medicine,
Department of General Internal Medicine, Yale University
Honorary Associate Professor, Medical Ethics and Law,
Faculty of Health Sciences and Medicine, Bond University (Australia)
Lecturer and Law and Ethics Lead,
School of Medicine, Keele University (UK)

and

ROBERT ROHRBAUGH MD

Professor of Psychiatry
Deputy Chair for Education and Career Development,
Department of Psychiatry
Director, Office of International Medical Student Education
Yale University

Radcliffe Publishing
London • New York

Radcliffe Publishing Ltd
33-41 Dallington Street
London EC1V 0BB
United Kingdom

www.radcliffepublishing.com

Electronic catalogue and worldwide online ordering facility

© 2011 Roger Worthington and Robert Rohrbaugh

Roger Worthington and Robert Rohrbaugh have asserted their right under the Copyright, Designs and Patents Act 1998 to be identified as the authors of this work.

All rights reserved. No part of this publication may be reproduced, stored in a retrieval system or transmitted in any form or by any means, electronic, mechanical, photocopying, recording or otherwise, without the prior permission of the copyright owner.

British Cataloguing in Publication Data

A catalogue record for this book is available from the British Library.

ISBN-13: 978 184619 310 1

The paper used for the text pages of this book is FSC certified. FSC® (The Forest Stewardship Council®) is an international network to promote responsible management of the world's forests.

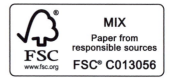

MIX
Paper from
responsible sources
FSC® C013056

Typeset by KnowledgeWorks Global Ltd, Chennai, India
Cover design by Cox Design Ltd, Witney, UK
Printed and bound by TJI Digital, Padstow, Cornwall, UK

Contents

Foreword

The authors of *Health Policy and Ethics* believe that something fundamental about the ethical values of a society can be learned by understanding its health policies. Through the use of several examples from various societies, they demonstrate the point nicely. We can learn much about our values by examining our healthcare policies and professional standards. Perhaps even more importantly, however, it is essential that those who create policy ensure that this thesis is true. That is, it is essential that our health policies (indeed all of our public policies) reflect our values and priorities. This is not a simple matter, and as various options are considered and various moral arguments are brought to bear in the development of health-care policy and professional standards, sound ethical analysis is needed. To best accomplish this, ethicists must have a seat at the table.

Though much of the terminology is relatively new, medical ethics has been a subject of consideration and scholarship since antiquity, and has informed medical practice for as long. The past several decades, however, have seen a great expansion of scholarship in this field, and it is now considered an essential part of the medical school curriculum. It is widely accepted within the medical profession that one cannot and should not practice medicine without grounding in at least the fundamentals of medical ethics. And, given the complexity of many of the questions we physicians now face, it is increasingly accepted among our profession that ethicists have something valuable to contribute. As we navigate the difficult waters of medical care, their insight and analyses of the difficult questions often prove helpful. As regional, national, and even international health policy continue to play an increasing role in the delivery of health care, it is essential that those crafting the policies reach the same understanding about the value of ethical analysis.

Healthcare policy has been a major subject of controversy in many places for many years. In the United States, at the time of this writing, it has been at the very forefront of our national conversation for years. Complex problems are unlikely to lend themselves to easy solutions. A thoughtful approach requires input from those with expertise in economics, medicine, nursing, law, politics, life sciences, research, history, epidemiology, technology and yes, ethics. In *Health Policy and Ethics* the authors provide an excellent illustration as to how an understanding of ethics can inform the ongoing development of health policy. They also show the value of a broad, global perspective. By considering the history and current status of health-care and medical ethics in cultures from China to Italy, and many others, we reach a better understanding of things both there and here (wherever 'here' happens to be for the reader).

While physicians are mindful that ethical analysis is often essential with regard to individual patient decisions, we also recognize that ethically sound decisions on an individual level can be greatly augmented, or be negated, by policy decisions made on a regional or national level. The basic premise of *Health Policy and Ethics* is that including ethical analysis will lead to more effective and successful policies. This seems clearly to be so. We need to understand what we truly value before we can effectively establish priorities. And, as this book nicely illustrates, it often proves interesting and helpful to consider what others value, and what others have done, even if we choose a different path.

As the authors have shown, examination of professional standards and policy can facilitate analysis of ethical issues in healthcare. Conversely, ethical analysis can and should inform ongoing policy development. Policies should be continually assessed in light of societal values through ethical analysis, and something akin to John Rawls' reflective equilibrium should continually be sought; when our policies are found to be inconsistent with our principles, one or the other (or perhaps both) should be revised. Ethical analysis in this domain is not easy, as things held sacred will at times conflict, and of course within a given society there will be variability in values and priorities between individuals and over time. The anticipated difficulties serve to further emphasize that the ongoing ethical analysis should include input from those with experience and skill at that task. This book successfully demonstrates that point. In addition, *Health Policy and Ethics* is a welcome bridge between these two fields, and a very worthwhile read for individuals whose primary interest lies in either one.

Mark R. Mercurio, M.D., M.A.
Director, Program for Biomedical Ethics
Yale University School of Medicine

About the authors

Roger P. Worthington, MA, Ph.D.

Roger Worthington is an Assistant (Adjunct) Professor of Medicine at Yale University (USA), and Honorary Associate Professor of Medical Ethics and Law at Bond University (Australia) leads on health care law and ethics at Keele University School of Medicine (UK). He co-runs a student exchange program between Keele and Yale with Robert Rohrbaugh; he works as an adviser in the public sector and provides continuing medical education and training programmes for the National Health Service (NHS) and he is a former consultant at the General Medical Council (UK). His MA in medical ethics is from Keele, and his doctorate in philosophy is from the State University of New York at Buffalo.

Robert M. Rohrbaugh, MD

Robert Rohrbaugh is Professor of Psychiatry and Deputy Chair for Education and Career Development in the Department of Psychiatry at Yale University School of Medicine. He also directs the Office of International Medical Student Education where he oversees the global health curriculum, develops international clinical electives for Yale students and brings international students to Yale for clinical electives. He consults to the Xiangya School of Medicine in Changsha China on the development of post-graduate medical education programs. His medical doctorate is from Yale University.

Contributors

Noor Sulastry Yurni Ahmad (Ph.D.)
Senior Lecturer, Department of Anthropology and Sociology
University of Malaya, Malaysia

Caroline Broughton (BDS, BSc, MB, ChB)
Foundation Doctor
University Hospital of North Staffordshire
Stoke-on-Trent, UK

Kwok-Yin Chan (BSc, MB, ChB)
Foundation Doctor
New Cross Hospital
Wolverhampton, UK

Jaazzmina Hussain (MB, ChB)
Foundation Doctor
Kettering General Hospital
Northamptonshire, UK

Sarah A. Lee (BSc, MD)
Anaesthesiology Resident
Massachusetts General Hospital
Boston, USA

Anthony Marfeo (BSc, MD)
Psychiatry Resident
Harvard University
Boston, USA

Carla Marienfeld (MD)
Psychiatry Resident
Department of Psychiatry
Yale University

Maya G. Prabhu (MSc, MD, LLB)
Psychiatry Resident
Department of Psychiatry
Yale University

PART 1

CHAPTER 1

Introduction

The basic provision of health care services is not something that can be taken for granted, and the extent to which patients are able to access services that they need, when and where they need them varies greatly between and within countries. Health care services, of whatever standard, cannot be provided in an ethical vacuum. While health policy debate is normally dominated by political and economic considerations, there is a moral dimension to the provision of health care, which can profoundly affect the care patients receive as well as the clinical outcomes. It is our belief, therefore, that ethical considerations need to be consciously factored into public policy considerations.

There is a growing recognition that health policy is not value neutral, and as a subject it cannot be regarded as an "ethics free zone." Leathard and McLaren describe how ethics is increasingly taking a key position in publications on health and social care;[1] Dawson and Verweij note that within bioethics, public health ethics is developing into a sub-discipline of its own,[2] and Hester describes how ethical deliberation and good public health practice are intrinsically part of good professional practice.[3] Murray notes in relation to the health reform program in the USA that:

> "There is a broad range of values that we want our health care system to embody and pursue—not just liberty but also justice and fairness, responsibility, medical progress, privacy, and physician integrity, among others."[4]

This is a tall order, perhaps, but they are important issues that ought to be actively discussed, and in this work we go on to say that being deprived of access to quality and affordable health services can put lives at risk, reduce life-expectancy, and impact on the quality of life of both individuals and populations.

Health care policies determine how health care is provided, and our thesis is that by analyzing health law, health policy and professional standards, something essential about the ethical values espoused by any given society can be revealed. In some countries, financial gain is a preeminent driving force behind the provision of health services, while in others what matters most is simple human survival, and in between these two extremes is a range of social and political models for delivering health care. Ethics is no optional extra within the policy arena, and when the sustainability of human life itself is at stake, the moral dimension to the provision of health care is always present, even if it is not recognized.

In short, our argument is that it is a matter of public interest to make room for serious ethical debate within the context of analyzing and determining health policy. An essential part of this analysis is examining critically the relation between what is legal and what is ethical, and we do not subscribe to the view that they are necessarily one and the same. This area of jurisprudence needs to be considered if ethics and policy are to work closer together. Integrating ethics into health policy discussion may not be achievable unless there is clarity as regards legal frameworks that are applicable in a given setting, and we discuss these issues more fully in the next chapter.

Ethics does not simply deal with abstractions—it can be used as a sharply analytic tool leading to practical suggestions for change. While barriers to change are sometimes physical and intensely practical, they are just as often conceptual and ideological. Effective policies have to be able to coordinate complex arrangements of organizations and services, and the provision of health care typically has to take account of large, diverse populations with different needs and preferences, and of necessity this renders the application of simple formulae near impossible.

Patient safety is an example of a specific issue where an ethical analysis can be useful. Patient safety is an increasingly important issue within systems of health care delivery, and this topic gives rise to policy considerations of their own that require ethical scrutiny. While health policies are not value-neutral, putting ethics and health policy within a single phrase is not something to which people are yet fully accustomed, and we argue that the linkage between these two domains is logical, significant and inescapable. While under Article 25 of the *United Nations Declaration of Human Rights* health is regarded as a fundamental human right, simply making this assertion does nothing to change the way things are in practice. Rights declarations have their place but effectively they serve as statements of intent; however, the possibility remains that rights-based claims to good quality care are morally defensible and worth close scrutiny.

External economic and political events play a significant part in the policy-making process, and addressing the underlying ethics and putting policies into perspective are important considerations. Improving health care service provision takes a great deal more than merely opening a hospital or spending additional resources. It requires sustained effort as well as an adequate supply of human and material resources in order for lasting improvements to be achieved, including simple access to basic services. Analyzing the ethical implications of health care policies governing efforts to change systems is critical to ensuring that policies are effective. Policies that contradict each other are doomed to fail, and we contend that these pitfalls can only be avoided if there is clarity of thinking and expression about the underpinning values.

Pragmatism and ethics need not work in opposition. Much will depend on how policies are formulated and how they relate to other policies, and often it is unclear who is making policy decisions according to what criteria. Policy confusion can ultimately lead to patients being harmed, for example, through lack of proper planning, and lack of access to necessary and appropriate treatments. Policy decision-making must reflect realities, but having no regard to the moral basis of health care provision makes it unlikely that anything resembling fair and equitable social arrangements will ever be achieved.

Health care policies to a greater or lesser extent reflect the collective values of society. Even in complex, socially diverse societies it is reasonable to suppose that some ethical values will be held in common, such as respect for patient autonomy, even though this concept may have different meanings for different people. The contention is that values change over time, they are not always made explicit, and they can vary significantly according to cultural and geographical context. Therefore, room must be made in a healthy society for reasonable accommodation towards a divergence of viewpoints, analysing the nature and scope of those values that are applicable to the provision of health services.

While there is ongoing debate about ethics and the global dimensions of public health,[5] little effort is generally expended in terms of analyzing the moral values behind health care. Significant differences exist between one country and another when it comes to being able to access quality, affordable health care in a timely manner. This is why we think that insights can be gained from looking at different countries in terms of how they deal with these issues. In this book we choose an international perspective to demonstrate that ethical analysis of health care policy in international settings offers a useful tool for exploring the values that underpin the provision of health care, and we go on and attempt to consider practical implications in terms of patient care.

Many obstacles to the effective provision of health care services exist, and these will have different characteristics in different national and international settings. Accessing health care in rural China, for instance, is a different proposition from accessing care in rural India or in the jungle areas of Malaysia, and it is certainly quite different from accessing health care in urban settings that have good, centralized systems for the provision of services.

OUTLINE

This book comprises three parts. *Part 1* sets out the theoretical, analytic framework for policy decision-making, providing an overview of health policy analysis and a rationale for the book as a whole. It examines relationships between law, health care and ethics, and different frameworks that can be used in policy analysis. These chapters are based mainly on frameworks and events relating to the UK. Firstly, when theoretical discussion takes place in the abstract it is difficult to make the leap from theory to practice and it is the intention of the authors that this book will have practical value. Secondly, in order to see if and how alternative frameworks might apply to important issues such as rationing or macro policy decision-making, there needs to be a fact basis upon which to build the arguments.

The British National Health Service (NHS) has many peculiar characteristics, and without first-hand experience, either as a provider or as a consumer of services, many features of the system might appear strange, even irrational. That may be, and it is argued in Chapter 4 that like ethics, logic is not a dominant feature in policy debate. The government in immediate post-war World War II Britain undertook a bold experiment in universal coverage, one that has survived (more or less intact) for over 60 years. Dramatic change has taken place with the health service; nonetheless, for good or bad the NHS has a uniqueness that in and of itself makes it interesting in terms of moral policy analysis. Papers in the second part of the book are for the most part not UK-based. It would be impossible to be truly global within the confines of a single volume; however, in *Part 2*, short chapters address different countries with a variety of different health care systems that collectively serve to illustrate: a) the nature of some of the problems encountered in providing health care services, b) something about the social values pertaining to those countries, and (c) the usefulness of an ethical component to the policy analysis.

CHAN AND MARIENFELD ON CHINESE ETHICS AND HEALTH CARE

Readers may be familiar with some of the ethical principles commonly employed in the West when analyzing clinical cases. But these are not the only types of ethical reasoning, and this chapter outlines some of the Chinese philosophies that have helped shape health policy decision-making in China. These ethical principles are of ancient Confucian origin, but they are not disconnected from modern medical practice, even if they need adapting in order to be of use in facing modern challenges. This chapter explores links between ancient and modern philosophies and health care practice and considers how Chinese health care has managed to stay relatively close to its philosophical roots.

Pressures arising on account of rapid social, political and economic change have meant the need to adapt, and there is evidence to suggest that the ancient principles are especially challenged in trying to meet the health care needs of growing and increasingly urbanized populations. These challenges are exemplified well by the case example of a young man and his family attempting to access care in connection with the onset of a psychotic disorder.

WORTHINGTON ON ETHICS AND PROFESSIONALISM IN MODERN INDIA

This chapter similarly looks to the past in order to understand some of the issues facing health care professionals, this time in present-day India. India also has rich

philosophical traditions, and yet this complex nation is slowly becoming disconnected from its own philosophical roots. This has a direct bearing on the way that
medicine is practiced, and while Western models of health care delivery are being
adopted in India, unlike in the West ethics and professionalism are rarely taught in
medical schools, and the legal and ethical frameworks of medical practice are not
well defined. If they are defined, then the mechanisms to uphold them are weak,
and standards of professionalism are being seriously challenged from commercial
pressures and more widely from evolving social change. In the past these values
were not necessarily made explicit because it was not considered necessary to do so;
they were considered an intrinsic part of everyday traditional culture. That situation,
however, no longer applies.

In most countries, there are significant differences in health care provision for
urban and rural populations, and India is no exception. Large sections of the rural
population have only limited access to medical care, and sometimes the only way
that people living in remote regions can access services is by travelling long distances and waiting to be seen in the poorly funded state-run hospitals. This chapter
includes an account of some of these difficulties, especially the implications that
arise in the context of rural health care in the Himalayas. A case example involving
a mother who is experiencing a difficult birth offers a poignant example.

AHMAD ON HEALTH POLICY DEVELOPMENTS IN MALAYSIA

Health care in Malaysia has some particular characteristics that make it an interesting example to study in terms of health policy trends. It operates within a fairly sta-
ble political environment, which means that unlike most other countries, long-term
policy planning is a "norm." Current trends, however, mean that a private sector is
becoming increasingly dominant, and in order to avoid restricting access to health
care, insurance-based solutions are now being sought.

This needs to be viewed against a political background where state health care
provision enjoys wide public support. Change, however necessary, is never easy,
and no one in Malaysia wants to give up on universal access. But as in other countries, this is coming under significant economic pressure. Another characteristic
is the urban-rural divide that, while it is not new, is tending to result in greater
inequalities of service provision, especially in the remote and isolated jungle areas
of the country. This has particular implications for women's health, which is a topic
of special focus. Also worth noting is the way the country deals with the issue of
cultural diversity. Islam is the dominant religious culture, influencing both legal
and social frameworks. However, sizeable minorities exist, such as the Indian and
Chinese communities, and the country's approach to multiculturalism offers clues
to how it has succeeded in maintaining social stability over time. In turn, this influences health policy decision-making, and this chapter provides added breadth to
the more general discussion about health care ethics and policy.

HUSSAIN AND BROUGHTON ON RELATIONS BETWEEN THE PHARMACEUTICAL INDUSTRY AND THE MEDICAL PROFESSION

The importance of linking theory and practice has already been described, and an area of health care with almost universal applicability is that concerning industry and its links with medicine. The influence of pharmaceutical companies on health care provision is well established and reaches all around the globe. It affects the way in which new drugs are researched and how much people pay for the medicines they need, as well as who has access to them. This chapter focuses on two aspects of a relationship that exists between commercial companies and medical professionals.

This relationship became the focus of considerable media attention in the USA in 2008 after evidence came to light of industry having had much closer financial ties with medicine than people had previously realized. Medical research and continuing medical education are respectively the focus of the two halves of a chapter that critically examines ethical arguments around conflict of interest. While these studies are based on examples from the USA, the moral arguments may not be so different elsewhere. Conflicts of interest can significantly (if indirectly) put patients at risk, for instance, in cases where a doctor's primary duty of care is compromised by undisclosed or partly disclosed financial ties with industry. Central to the thesis of this book is the concept that moral values have an impact on patient care, which is something that this chapter particularly seeks to illustrate.

PRABHU ON THE ROLE OF PHYSICIANS IN THE DETENTION CENTER AT GUANTANAMO BAY, CUBA

This chapter has a different focus in that it is concerned with the detention of "enemy aliens" from the US wars in Iraq and Afghanistan, and in particular with what has been happening at Guantanamo Bay. This whole operation could not have been carried out without the participation and compliance of trained, practicing clinicians. The legal and ethical basis under which the Guantanamo detention center functions provides vivid examples of professionalism in practice in what can be described as a perverse and highly challenging setting. Legal and ethical frameworks were not totally ignored; rather they were re-interpreted in order to try and justify practices that many regard as indefensible. Doctors may be trained to serve, but whom and how they serve must come under constant scrutiny if society wishes to try and prevent a recurrence of some horrors from the past.

Among the human rights and legal issues is the participation of medical professionals in utilizing "enhanced interrogation techniques" in order to obtain information considered pertinent to protecting the USA and facilitating militarily defined goals. The techniques used are critically examined in this chapter, as is the relationship with torture. US policy after 9/11 is examined, along with rationales for reneging on longstanding international commitments and legal conventions.

LEE ON PATIENT PERCEPTIONS OF RISK AND THE IMPLICATIONS FOR POLICY

This chapter addresses a different type of risk from one of international security. Here the topic is pertinent to health policy debate because the subject of risk is not always properly understood. It is something many people think they understand, yet everyone approaches it in slightly different ways. Patient perceptions of risk have a direct bearing on the way that decisions are made, either to agree or refuse to take part in medical research or to undergo treatment and diagnostic procedures. This applies to individual episodes of patient care as well as to macro policy decision-making. Public policy towards risk is sometimes so focused on risk avoidance that it misses the point, in that risk can actually be "an enabler." Without taking risks, change does not happen, and too much risk avoidance can lead to excessive caution, whereby policy makers are prevented from taking effective action. This applies to many aspects of public policy but has a particular relevance to health care in that it concerns decisions made by individual patients and clinicians, as well as by governments.

Clinicians normally address risk from a rational, science-based perspective as a result of their prior training, and this can sometimes be at odds with more person-centered approaches to medicine that increasingly feature in modern medical practice, especially in the West. Sometimes doctors hold irrational views, and the same can apply to human subjects as well as patients; some difficulties are about communication but others are more conceptual, which necessarily include ethical and legal frameworks. While the author writes from a UK perspective, the issues that she addresses are much broader in terms of their application.

MARFEO ON ELECTROCONVULSIVE THERAPY AND ITALIAN HEALTH CARE

This chapter has a European focus and is written against the context of the Italian *Servizio Sanitario Nazionale* (SSN). While it considers legal and ethical frameworks that are used in health policy decision-making in Italy, the author draws some interesting comparisons with the British NHS. In terms of clinical focus, the chapter discusses the controversial use of electroconvulsive therapy. Over the past half-century there have been several changes with regards to scientific and popular acceptability (or not) towards this therapy. The chapter sits well alongside the chapter on risk in that here the ethical and policy frameworks are about a form of therapy that is considered high-risk but effective. Italian public opinion has not always been consistent towards this controversial therapy, and the conclusions drawn are interesting and informative. They are likely to have applications in other national settings, both in terms of public policy towards the therapy itself and on the amount of attention paid more generally towards public attitude, scientific risk, social policy and medicine.

Part 3 has just one chapter that focuses on comparative analysis. It is designed to enable readers to look at the examples of health policy in action, to consider some of the implications, and to identify common strands for shared understanding. This analysis has the potential for improving the quality of health policy decision-making, which in turn should lead to improved access to affordable services.

Better policy can lead to an increase in respect for people's individual and collective rights and responsibilities towards health care service provision. Asking questions and defining problems is one thing, but more important perhaps is being able to find ways of viewing health policy that can help to improve patient outcomes. Policy analysis is a matter of purely academic debate if it does not engage directly with patient care. Because health policy focuses on complex issues that non-specialists may find hard to understand, it is sometimes considered "the preserve of the few". It ought not to be that way, and this concluding part to the book seeks to identify common strands, to explore points of intersection, and to highlight issues about equality and diversity. It is hoped that overall this analysis will be of value to all those who are interested in health policy for the future.

REFERENCES

1. Leathard A, McLaren S. *Ethics: Contemporary Challenges in Health and Social Care.* Bristol, England: Policy Press; 2007.
2. Dawson A, Verweij M. *Ethics, Prevention, and Public Health: issues in biomedical ethics.* Oxford, England: Clarendon Press; 2007.
3. Boylan M, editor. *Public Health Policy and Ethics.* New York, NY: Springer; 2005.
4. Murray TH. *American values and health care reform. New Eng. J. Med.* December 23, 2009. Available at: www.nejm.org/doi/full/10.1056/NEJMp0911116 (accessed April 6, 2011).
5. Dawson, op. cit.

CHAPTER 2

Why ethics and health policy

RATIONALE

Ethics does not regularly feature in health policy discussion, and while there may be exceptions to the rule, this represents an important omission. This chapter endeavours to explain the theory behind why we maintain that health policy should actively incorporate ethical perspectives, and why if this were to happen, policies would have a greater degree of social validity and effectiveness. Economic and political considerations normally dominate discussions about health policy determination. This is a "norm," and it is not surprising that policies that determine the manner in which health care is delivered are subject to such practical constraints. But this two-dimensional approach towards setting health policy has significant limitations, and incorporating ethics as the third dimension is both necessary and expedient.

Ethics is the term normally used within the context of professional discourse, but application alone does not succeed in differentiating one term from another; ethics and morals are in effect synonymous, the first simply being derived from the Greek and the second from the Latin. A "moral" is essentially a social more, or custom; it can therefore change with time and it can change in relation to different geographical, cultural and legal settings. (For a fuller discussion on these issues, notably in the context of global health education, *see* Anderson F, Wanson T, 2009).[1]

MORAL VALUES

A range of moral values manifests itself in different cultures and societies at different points in time. But this does not preclude the existence or exploration of commonly held beliefs and ethical standards. On the contrary, things only tend to be problematic when there is insistence on framing ethical discussion in relation to moral absolutes, classing anything else as moral relativism and to be avoided at all costs. Arguments between attachment to absolutes and the rejection of relativism are not especially helpful, whereas the notion that a society can decide for itself concerning acceptable or unacceptable standards is altogether more interesting. Society can decide such things irrespective of belief in moral absolutes. Moral absolutes may or may not exist, but if they do exist this book could be taken up in explaining why some might be "in" and others "out." Overall they are to be treated with considerable caution.

The fact that in a pluralist society there are many different ways of viewing matters pertaining to life, death and standards of behavior is proof that there is more than one way of dealing with moral problems. It is too easy to stifle argument, saying "well, that is a matter of moral absolutes." Something may be an absolute for protagonists of one cause, but the exact opposite could be considered absolute by protagonists from a different cause. Deciding who is right and wrong on a moral issue to some extent presupposes that matters can be viewed in black or white, and moral/ethical arguments are rarely that clear.

Another way of deciding things could be by reference to external sources seen as having moral weight and authority, such as international agencies or legal authorities. This, coupled with the individual exercise of moral judgment, seems to be a valid way of reaching difficult decisions. While some commonalities inevitably exist between different cultural traditions, cultural groups nonetheless reference their ideals in different ways, both in terms of language and modes of expression, which adds another layer of complexity. If moral values are not to be viewed in a vacuum, they require a level of engagement that must go beyond abstract philosophical debate.

Philosophical discourse has a tendency to approach issues in a way that some would say is inaccessible to the general public, and a pragmatic approach towards addressing ethics and policy is perhaps what is needed. If issues are handled appropriately, then even the most controversial topics can be addressed. While substantive issues can and should provoke lively debate, taking an inclusive stance is usually an effective way of avoiding ideological, fundamentalist bias.

PERSONAL BELIEF

The difficult subject of religion is sometimes avoided in ethical discourse, but in 2008 it provided the focus of attention when for the first time the General Medical Council in the UK issued guidance on *Personal Beliefs and Medical Practice*.[2] This wisely limits itself to giving higher level advice on how to deal with issues that give rise to conflict, rather than stating what someone should or should not do in a given situation. However, it actively encourages moral engagement, and in the wider context of debates about health policy, society surely is weakened if its moral values are simply ignored.

A mature society needs to debate these issues and to consider, for example, whether standards and codes of practice are thought to be binding:
1 by reason of being encapsulated in law
2 because a public authority such as a regulatory or government agency asserts that they reflect a body of opinion

3   because they are aspirational and set a standard to which people sometimes fail to live up but which nonetheless matter
4   because they set a basic minimum below which anything else is unacceptable
5   because they are customary and the way things have always been, and so by definition do not need to change.

STANDARD SETTING

Standard setting may involve more than one of these descriptors, but no process can embrace them all because they contain contradictory premises. Point one above may be stating a fact but on its own is not a moral argument; points two, three and four have some moral validity but they need to be weighed one against another, and point five makes assumptions that do not even admit to the possibility of change, and may therefore tend to stifle rather than stimulate debate.

It is common for difficult cases involving disputes about medical decision-making to be arbitrated in court, and for at least some of the arguments employed in adjudication, especially at appellate level, to be moral, i.e. framed by reference to ethical standards. Just as in setting ethical standards one has to be cognisant of the law to avoid recommending someone to behave in a way that is contrary to the law, similarly, making a legal determination requires an awareness of what society thinks is morally acceptable. This implies no circularity because ethics and law occupy different domains and have slightly different functions. What needs exploring is when, where and how they intersect.

The majority of the time, maintaining ordinary standards of practice is a necessary and sufficient condition that demonstrates meeting minimum legal standards. This normative definition of standards is sufficient to protect most patients most of the time from unnecessary, avoidable medical harm. Acceptable, realistic and achievable standards of practice exist within a range that may *include* best practice, although not as a matter of necessity because circumstances do not always permit. If doctors function at a level whereby they merely avoid clinical negligence or serious professional misconduct, they may avoid trouble but it would be difficult for them to achieve best practice. Clinicians sometimes argue that best practice ethical standards are unrealistic and unachievable; however, if reasonably defined that should not be the case.

LAW VERSUS ETHICS

A dynamic relationship exists between ethics and law, but to see one as being coterminous with the other presupposes a view of the world framed by moral absolutes; i.e., prior to non-negotiable. If, on the other hand, ethics and law were considered to be completely detached from one another, that would imply that somebody could potentially put him- or herself above the law simply by invoking a moral argument.

While that could be the case if a particular law is considered "unjust," the important question here is how the two domains called "law" and "ethics" interrelate.

Plato and Aristotle both wrestled with this problem and so it is not new, and it would be foolish to suppose that these complex matters can be settled within the space of a few pages. However, in the context of health policy and ethics, the nature of the relationship between ethics and law is pivotal in terms of being able to do meaningful and effective analysis.

Sometimes writers refer to an ethical dilemma, as if that were akin to doing ethical analysis, which is clearly is not the case any more than inserting a few ethical terms into a text, such as simple references to ethical principles, constitutes a moral argument. Meaningful ethical discussion requires attention to detail, and making a critical examination of underlying concepts. This can be done without categorizing each element in relation to autonomy, beneficence, non-maleficence or justice—the so-called four ethical principles. Asking a series of questions is not enough, and it is a poor substitute for expending intellectual and sometimes emotional energy in finding a solution capable of working in real-life situations.

We have limited faith in the four principles when it comes to finding workable solutions to real, practical problems. There is benefit to be had from talking about a problem, and it is conceivable that a solution can be found in this way; however, in many instances, the demands of one principle are in conflict with the demands of another, which is the reason why their "true" place (if one exists) lies within ethical discourse, and not problem-solving and analytic decision-making.

PERTINENT COMMON LAW

Examining some legal cases may help in clarifying the extent of the interrelationship between law and ethics. For example, in the case of *Gillick v. West Norfolk and Wisbech Area Health Authority*, 1985, there are several references to the significance of social values. As Lord Templeman says: "Social issues need not finally be determined and are not best determined by lawyers or by doctors."[3] This is a direct and helpful statement to the effect that a court is not the proper place for defining ethical standards. However, this does not prevent judges from citing ethical guidance in an opinion. Ethics informs the law, and the law informs ethics, but they work in different ways, and while they can point in the same direction, that does not make one mode of reasoning dependent on the other. Interdependence and interactions are better ways of characterizing this relationship.

The legal validity of ethical guidance was subject to scrutiny on one notable occasion. The case of *Oliver Burke v. the General Medical Council (UK)* started in 2004, soon after the General Medical Council (UK) (GMC) issued guidance on *Withholding and Withdrawing Life-prolonging Treatment*. The guidance was challenged and taken to judicial review, and when the case was decided, the court first came to a view that aspects of the guidance were indeed unlawful. However, judgment was overturned on appeal the following year, and Lord Philips gave public endorsement to the guidance. He went so far as to say that it "should be understood and implemented at every level throughout the National Health Service and throughout the medical profession."[4] This endorsement of an ethical standard, set independently of government, was unusual and it led to an educational campaign to help to make the guidance better known and understood.[5]

While this case shows courts making reference to and scrutinizing ethical standards, the other half of the equation concerns drafting guidance and the way in which it draws upon the law. As a case in point, the GMC issued guidance in 2007 for doctors treating patients under the age of 18.[6] It had not previously issued guidance for this group of patients, and this departure from previous practice was in part prompted by a change in the law;[7] the guidance contains an appendix citing reference to both primary legislation and case law, and the GMC conducted a review to ensure that the new guidance would be compliant with the law. This drafting process included a period of public consultation, and as a consequence of this the guidance reflects a wide body of opinion. Therefore, while it can be seen that the law influences the drafting of ethical guidance, it does not seek to determine the content. Hence, whichever starting point you choose, law and ethics coexist and interact, but while performing different functions.

To take a further example, the GMC issues guidance on decision-making and consent, and in 2008 the guidance on this topic was substantially updated. This was in no small way due to changes in the law, such as the Mental Capacity Act (2005) that made provision for advance refusals of treatment and the appointment of "donees", or health proxies that hitherto were not part of the legal framework in England and Wales. Case (common) law had also moved forward since previous guidance on consent was issued, and the model being upheld by the courts was more patient-centered than it had been previously.

All of these changes were reflected in the new, updated guidance. However, once guidance is issued by a statutory body such as the GMC, it assumes a measure of legal validity, such that if a doctor deviates significantly away from these standards s/he can expect to be reprimanded and/or to have to provide an explanation. Disciplinary proceedings are only quasi judicial hearings, but if a doctor is investigated and deemed unfit to practice medicine, the right to appeal is heard in the High Court. Furthermore, if a negligence case were to be made in court against an individual doctor, it would be to GMC ethical guidance that lawyers would look to help them define the reasonable expectations that patients should have of their doctor. (The process of standards-setting and investigation has significant public and patient involvement.) Hence, the process is entirely two-way; the law no more works in isolation than ethical standards are determined without reference to the law.

RISK

To illustrate this further it is worth considering how courts approach the concept of risk. Risk is something that is difficult to quantify and has different meanings to different people in different situations. A patient, for example, may consider a remote risk of suffering minor harm resulting from a medical intervention as something trivial and easily justified if offset by the anticipated benefits. However, another patient wanting the same procedure might think differently and want to know every detail before making a decision, and even then withhold his or her consent.

Things do not stop there, because risks may be significant for other reasons. Risk may be remote in terms of probability but serious and significant in terms of outcome; for instance, in situations where, if things go wrong, the consequence is catastrophic and results in the death of a patient. However, at the other extreme, a complication could be very likely to happen but be minor in its effect, e.g. a headache resulting from an epidural given during labor. In between these extremes is a continuum of possibilities, and clinicians sometimes look for guidance on how best to deal with these kinds of issues. This may stem from the genuine desire to do the best for patients, or it may reflect a more minimalist approach, wanting to ensure that no claims for negligence are likely to ensue. The first standard is patient-centered, the second is physician-centered, and reflects a difference in attitude.

Arguments about risk have been debated at length in the courts. For example, a landmark case in Australia focused on standards used by doctors to communicate risk to patients when seeking their consent,[8] and an English case settled in the House of Lords adjudicated on a similar point.[9] Both cases considered reasonableness in terms of what a patient could and should expect from a clinician in terms of the amount of information provided to enable a patient to make a meaningful decision about whether or not to give consent. In both instances surgery was for an elective procedure, the first for an eye problem and the second for a low back problem, neither of which was life-threatening. In both cases the patient suffered an adverse result that could have been foreseen but that nonetheless had not been anticipated. The surgeons in question failed to provide a warning about these potential but unlikely adverse outcomes, and the fact that these cases went to the highest court before a final determination was given is an indication of the complexity surrounding these issues.

Risk is a social construct and not an exact science, and if people do not take risks they are not able to lead normal, meaningful lives (for instance, nobody would ever get into a car), so the problem effectively has to do with necessity and proportion. Therefore, if a risk is unavoidable, can anything be done to minimize the consequences if things go wrong? And if a risk is avoidable, what reasonable alternative courses of action exist that might achieve the same or a similar result, e.g. the relief of pain or an improved chance of survival? Ultimately, only patients can make this kind of decision (if they have legal capacity) by factoring in personal preferences and priorities along with the clinical advice.

Nonetheless, it is the doctor who has to know what ethical and legal standard to apply in the course of doing his or her job, which brings the discussion back to the need for guidance, and to finding a workable way of dealing with problems such as risk. Some institutions (and some people) are more risk-aware or more risk-averse than others, and because in medicine bad judgment can make the difference between life and death, this is not something that can be overlooked.

EVERYDAY PRACTICE

In terms of ethical standards in everyday clinical practice, it is clear that the law defines the minimum standard and does not usually try and stipulate best practice. Firstly, the courts may not know what that entails; it is the clinician who has to interpret and apply standards in the context of his/her own knowledge and skills and the needs of each patient. Secondly, the law is there as a measure of protection and/or last resort, and not a way to micro-manage normal everyday activity. The implication here is that:

- low, minimal thresholds set standards below which a reasonable practicing professional ought not to fall
- upper thresholds indicate best practice standards to which conscientious clinicians can and should aspire
- in between these two standards is a continuum in which much routine clinical activity takes place.

A regulatory body has to decide where to pitch its guidance, and aiming for the top would mean recognizing that most of the time this standard may not reasonably be attainable. Aiming low means expressing everything in negative terms, stating which standards are unacceptable and which ones would call into question a doctor's right to practice.[10] In the UK, the Bolam judgment of 1957[11] set the basic standard for clinical negligence for over half a century, advocating a standard defined by reference to what a reasonable local body of professional opinion considered acceptable. While it provided a reasonable comfort zone for doctors, it was never patient-centered, and subsequent test cases succeeded in broadening the scope of the test for reasonableness.[12,13]

JURISPRUDENCE

There is a significant and relevant body of literature about the content and function of law. Because relationships between ethics and law play such a significant part in the theory underpinning this book, they need to be explored further. As Hart says in his famous book *The Concept of Law*:

> "It is in no sense a necessary truth that laws reproduce or satisfy certain demands of morality, though in fact they have often done so."[14]

In these short lines the whole basis of legal systems can be called into question; most modern liberal democracies have adopted systems of law derived from positivist legal traditions, and one of the tenets of legal positivism is that it is not a necessary condition for law to be based on a system of morality, even if law from time to time employs moral arguments. This is consistent with the explanations given above.

The problem of linking legal and moral standards too closely is that such a union has unwanted implications. Hart was writing during the early 1960s when legal and social traditions were beginning to be seriously challenged. There were pressing issues of the day about morality and social order, and in 1962 Hart writes that:

> "It is surely clear that anyone who holds the question whether a society has the 'right' to enforce morality, or whether it is morally permissible for any society to enforce its morality by law, to be discussable at all, must be prepared to deploy some … general principles of critical morality."[15]

This is no doubt true, but the legal enforcement of morality is no small matter. For instance, if there is no enforcement of the law, the result at one extreme is a state of anarchy. At the other extreme, if the enforcement of morality is performed with zeal the result is totalitarianism, which denies freedom of expression and individual human rights. Too much permissibility in society may be harmful, as too with over-regulation and enforcement. Both can have unintended consequences, and so an ethical goal is to try and find a balance between these extremes.

Extremes of viewpoint can lead to situations where, for example, in some countries, merely to be seen walking down the street with the wrong dress code could provide grounds for corporal punishment. Or, to take another example, under some legal systems having sexual relations outside marriage could result in a sentence of death, which demonstrates that questions of enforcement are not merely matters of philosophical debate. These matters have political overtones and they can influence an entire social order. Thus, the relationship between law and morality has a direct bearing on how people conduct their day-to-day lives, on how law is administered by the authorities, and on how standards of personal and professional morality are viewed and upheld. Law and morality are not often debated in this way outside of universities, and even then in departments of law and philosophy more than medicine. But if ethical debate is going to play its part in a mature society, jurisprudence needs to be included within the terms of reference for weighing difficult decisions.

POLICY EXAMPLE

To take a practical example, policies on resuscitation vary between institutions and between jurisdictions, and uncertainties about when to perform cardiopulmonary resuscitation and when not may reflect a sense of social unease about death as well as about the exercise of clinical judgment.[16] Coming to a settled view on an issue such as this is easier if the terms of reference are known and clearly described. These can be taken to include elements of moral as well as legal reasoning, and decisions around end-of-life tend to include both these elements.

If unwarranted or inappropriate cardiopulmonary resuscitation is undertaken, a dying patient could be subjected to repeated physical assaults as well as to assaults on their dignity. Fear of how the law might view a decision *not* attempt resuscitation is what tends to drive what some would regard as a futile attempt to "save life." If the law acknowledges the uncertainty that often surrounds this type of decision, it leaves sufficient room for ethical reasoning. Life and death may be a matter of black and white but the process of dying is not, and there is always room for moral reasoning, including and especially in the business of policy formulation.

PHILOSOPHY OF LAW

While there are some long-standing disputes that exist in relation to legal theory, which will not be discussed here, the background to legal theory has a potential to form part of normal ethical discourse. It forms a substratum that is capable of providing a rational, underpinning theoretical basis for ethical discussion. Philosophy of law has meaning and relevance in the messy world of modern medical practice. Medicine is messy in the sense that medicine is not an exact science and that there will always be differences of opinion, and messy in the political sense in terms of the different ways in which medicine is practiced. Discussion about moral and legal theory may seem a world away from the practical necessities of applying medical skill and expertise, but making decisions in situations where the fragility of human life is at stake provide examples of how theory can help to inform practice.

Legal philosophy includes inclusive and exclusive approaches to positivism as well, as natural law theory. (For a general account of legal positivism and the role it has played over time, *see* Murphy, 2005.)[17] Natural law theory tends to rely on some form of higher authority or external agency in order to determine what is right and wrong and provide the basis for maintaining law and order. The positivist view, on the other hand, leans towards the belief that society determines for itself the legal and moral standards that it wishes to apply. This leads one to debate social choice, social contracts and other kinds of social and political theory, which—interesting as they are—lie beyond the scope of this book.

POSITIVISM

In terms of the two types of positivism, an *exclusivist* approach seeks to avoid the circularity that arises from defining legal validity by referring to something that is itself hard to define, e.g. morals; at the same time it seeks to avoid relativism in legal and moral reasoning. But this is quite a difficult balance to try and achieve. A Kantian approach tends towards an exclusivist approach to positivism, whereas *inclusivist* interpretations of legal theory support the view that moral criteria are sometimes, but not always, necessary conditions for legal validity. In other words, they can offer proof of sufficiency when it comes to establishing legal validity. (The established way to differentiate between them is normally by making reference to legal convention and standards of normativity, which is known as the "rule of recognition").[18]

The inclusivist approach accords with a philosophy of law that is employed in this book. (For a fuller explanation, *see* Coleman, 2001.)[19] A related question that arises in connection with this approach to the function of law in society is how to define the role it plays in trying to correct an injustice, especially when it occurs within the context of medical negligence.

NEGLIGENCE

Negligence is not a helpful concept to use in terms of setting standards of professionalism, but it is still a relevant topic. The criteria for determining negligence generally require for there to be:
- a professional duty of care
- a breach of the professional duty of care
- the breach must result in harm being caused
- it must be established that harm was caused by the agent, i.e. the person(s) being sued
- it is for the plaintiff (complainant) to establish proof.

How society addresses questions of corrective justice determines what happens in the courts and who pays compensation to whom, an area in which considerable sums of money are paid out each year to settle medical cases. The principles of compensatory justice apply in different ways in different jurisdictions, and what matters here are the various attitudes adopted by society towards "righting wrongs." This reveals much about jurisprudence and the prevailing moral and legal order. We will continue to unpack some of these ideas.

JUSTICE AND PATIENT-CENTERED CARE

Patients can be harmed as a result of being denied care, and health policy that takes in the ethical dimension has the potential to influence patient outcomes. In essence, an ethical policy ought to be aimed at trying to deliver good quality *patient*-centered care. (This should be a truism, but health care providers often have other agendas.) If harm arises as a consequence of ordinary medical error, then no compensation would normally be considered. However, in a proven case of clinical negligence the situation changes, and when it comes to determining levels of compensation some important philosophical issues arise.

These have to do with attitudes to corrective and distributive justice, which reflect the prevailing social and moral values within a given society. The key issues are:

- who ultimately pays the compensation
- the legal and moral basis for paying compensation
- the intended end use of monies awarded
- if there is a punitive element, what this is meant to achieve
- whether the main beneficiary is the individual or the community
- and to what extent evidence of criminality or gross clinical negligence make a difference.

These are important topics, and in the context of a particular health care system they are revealing as reflections of the values system underlying the legal basis for paying compensation, or of attempting to "right a wrong." The first difficulty is that with health care claims it is often not possible fully to rectify a problem, and monetary payment is either just an acknowledgement that a wrong has been committed, or else it is a payout to try and mediate some of the long-term effects, such as additional costs of living, and/or from being unable to work. Causation is pivotal when it comes to attaching blame, but this is not the place for discussing theories of causation, or the role they play in determining negligence.

COMPENSATION AND BLAME

For compensation payments to be considered, blame normally has to be established, except in a no-fault legal system such as that of New Zealand, where both parties to a dispute share the cost of meeting a claim. For most out-of-court settlements, responsibility is not formally acknowledged, even though wronged individuals still receive monetary benefit. For example, it is easy for claimants in the UK seeking compensation from the NHS to compare the size of payouts to those made in a country such as the USA. But straightforward comparisons are not easy, and in the USA payments can be taken up very largely with paying medical bills, which is a situation that does not normally apply in the UK.

There are other questions that arise that deal with how widely risk is spread in terms of the size of the pool available to claimants, and it makes no sense to win a judgment that promises a settlement which in the end cannot be awarded. If risk is spread widely then the burden does not fall on any one person (or group of persons). If claims are made against the NHS, the pool potentially comprises all central taxpayer receipts, but in the private sector risk distribution is different and is underwritten by independent commercial entities; if there is a punitive element to a payment then the situation changes again. Punitive claims have an added component, which brings with it its own philosophical problems.

DAMAGES

There appears to be no clear and consistent rationale that judges use when making punitive awards in terms of "what kind of message is being sent and to whom." If a punitive award is made against the NHS then it could be argued that the patient is the just beneficiary but that government is the net loser in having to meet the claim. But it can also be argued that this represents a *benefit* to society because it is an efficient method of distributing risk, helping to raise standards. While the deterrent effect of reducing clinical negligence by having effective legal remedies is unproven, without access to such remedies patients might be that much more vulnerable. (In the UK there is a centralized system for dealing with complaints against the NHS, which operates as a separate authority under the name: *The National Health Service Litigation Authority, or NHSLA*).

A judge perhaps ought to state when making a punitive award whether the intention is to punish the wrongdoers, to provide incentives to raise standards of care, or simply to provide somebody with monies in excess of normal levels of compensation because of the amount of harm done and because there is no better way of righting that wrong. In truth, the intention is probably a mix of all three, and in cases of *gross* negligence, it is possible that a criminal action would have to be pursued against the person or persons responsible.

DISTRIBUTIVE JUSTICE

Other mechanisms exist for compensatory justice, or for distributing (or redistributing) burdens, risks and benefits within society. For instance, distributive justice is an ethical principle, and it can be utilized to help determine *how* resources are allocated to help promote general conditions of equity. It is essentially an expression of social justice, whereby fairness and social inclusion are the key concepts. However, another and appropriate term to use here would be "corrective justice," which lacks the political overtones inherent within the redistribution of assets. If the primary objective in making an award is to restore the *status quo ante*, then corrective justice is the better term to use. However, repairing human bodies is not the same as repairing property or motor vehicles, and so the matter is not settled.

It can be argued that corrective justice is a negative application of something that we call simply "justice," and that distributive justice is a more positive application of the term. However, the positive/negative distinction does not really hold because restoring a "wrongful" distribution to its "rightful" state necessarily implies making social and moral judgments. Ultimately, the fact cannot be ignored that in a medical setting it may be impossible to restore a pre-existing balance in terms of "social goods." (This term has often been used to encompass rights to health. *See* Rawls, 1999.)[20]

No amount of material compensation can bring back a life, or bring it back to the way it was, for instance, before a patient was rendered incontinent or paralyzed by the effects of a surgical intervention. This potentially calls into question the entire process of paying compensation in health-related claims. In addition, it presupposes that there is a large enough pool of assets to be used to bring about redistribution in paying out claims for compensation, and it also fails to address the basic issue of "who ultimately is paying whom for what." Medical negligence and questions of compensation are much more difficult than they might at first seem.

If it is not possible to restore a situation to what it was before, then it may be irrational for society to pay out large sums in compensation, especially when monies come from central taxation. On the other hand, that would seem to ignore the fact a person's life was changed by negligent actions of somebody else, and that a patient's quality of life is irreconcilably different from what it was before.

The real distinction to be made here is that a corrective duty of repair is retrospective, whereas redistributive elements of claims for compensation are prospective in nature. This distinction is more meaningful than the positive/negative distinction, and a moral duty of repair has elements that are both personal and collective. The negligent health professional owes the patient an apology, which is looking to past events, but at the same time, society acknowledges that the patient has been harmed and may need long-term emotional and physical support and assistance, which is evidently about looking forward and takes account of the moral as well as the legal element of responsibility.

The burden on individuals to cope with a life of sudden disability that came about through no fault of their own is considerable, and society has to acknowledge this as best it can, and to ignore such claims would represent a serious form of injustice. However, if the total number of claims relative to the amount of care provided overall rises year on year, this eventually means less money going into patient care. (As of March 31, 2008, "the NHSLA estimates that it has potential liabilities of £12.06 billion, of which £11.9 billion relate to clinical negligence claims," which represents a considerable drain on the public purse).[21] In other words, if a service provider, such a group of hospitals, raises standards with the specific intention of reducing the number of claims made, that could be of net benefit to society and to patients. However, if standards remain the same and accountants simply write down more money each year for meeting claims, then patients may not derive any benefit over the longer term, and the community as a whole suffers.

As matters of social policy it is important to consider how these different elements impact on health policies, and analysis of such issues ought to make future planning easier, or if not easier then at least better informed. It should now be clear why relating legal frameworks to ethical frameworks has a potential to bring about clarity of purpose in both defining standards of clinical practice as well as when clarifying the basis for paying out compensation.

OMBUDSMEN

There is one final branch of the law on compensation to consider, and the office of the ombudsman can play an interesting and significant part. In England it acts under a devolved authority from Parliament, and while its activities do not involve formal judicial processes, its investigations are nonetheless thorough, and its ensuing recommendations carry a degree of force. The outcome of an inquiry in which a health care organization is found to be at fault offers another example of a process aimed at trying to right a wrong, and Britain is just one country that makes use of the office of an ombudsman (a term that has no feminine, even if the post-holder is a woman).

One thing that is especially at stake is public confidence, and in conclusion, two key characteristics of this kind of process are worth noting. Firstly, before an ombudsman will open an investigation other avenues should have been exhausted in terms of having sought and failed to achieve satisfaction, e.g. from local governance arrangements and regulatory procedures. This means that in some cases, both a service provider and a public regulator may be at fault in terms of failing to provide good quality care and failing to respond adequately to patients' concerns.[22]

The second point is about principles, and in the UK ombudsmen adhere to a set of "Principles for Remedy" for conducting investigations and trying to remedy situations, in which either a proper explanation is owed or a formal apology, such as for a wronged patient or his or her bereaved relative, or else an amount of compensation. (This process is separate from that in which legal redress is sought and a patient tries to prove clinical negligence.) The aim of such inquiries is to restore public confidence in the system, and to protect the individual who has been a victim of poor service for which the State is ultimately responsible, while trying to ensure that similar failings do not happen in the future. The *Principles for Remedy* are: getting it right; being customer focused; being open and accountable; acting fairly and proportionately; putting things right; and seeking continuous improvement. These translate to mean:

- If possible, returning the complainant and, where appropriate, others who have suffered similar injustice or hardship to the position they would have been in if the maladministration or poor service had not occurred

- If that is not possible, compensating the complainant and such others appropriately
- Considering fully and seriously all forms of remedy (such as apology, an explanation, remedial action to prevent a recurrence, or financial compensation)
- Providing the appropriate remedy in each case.[23]

These principles provide a good end point to the discussion about principles of justice and the options open to patients when things do not go according to plan through either failings in systems of management, or failure on the part of an organization or individual to ensure patients receive good quality care.

REFERENCES

1. Anderson F, Wanson T. Beyond medical tourism: authentic engagement in global health. *Virtual Monitor.* 2009; **11**(7): 506–10.
2. General Medical Council (UK), 2008. *Guidance: personal beliefs and medical practice.* Available at: www.gmc-uk.org/guidance/ethical_guidance/personal_beliefs/personal_beliefs.asp (accessed August 12, 2009).
3. Gillick v. West Norfolk and Wisbech Area Health Authority, UKHL 7, 1985. Available at: www.bailii.org/uk/cases/UKHL/1985/7.html (accessed August 12, 2009).
4. Burke, R (on the application of) v. General Medical Council & Ors [2005] EWCA Civ 1003 §83. Available at: www.bailii.org/ew/cases/EWCA/Civ/2005/1003.html (accessed August 13, 2009).
5. General Medical Council (UK). *GMCtoday;* August, 2007. Previously available at: www.gmc-uk.org/publications/gmc_today/index.asp (accessed September 25, 2009).
6. General Medical Council (UK). *0–18 years: guidance for all doctors.* Available at: www.gmc-uk.org/guidance/ethical_guidance/children_guidance/index.asp (accessed August 13, 2009).
7. Children Act 2004. Available at: www.opsi.gov.uk/acts/acts2004/ukpga_20040031_en_1 (accessed August 13, 2009).
8. Rosenberg v. Percival, High Court of Australia (2001). Available at: www.ipsofactoj.com/international/2001/Part05/int2001(5)-005.htm (accessed August 13, 2009).
9. Chester v. Afshar, UKHL 41 (2004). Available at: www.bailii.org/uk/cases/UKHL/2004/41.html (accessed August 13, 2009).
10. General Medical Council (UK). Sanctions guidance (information for lawyers and others). www.gmc-uk.org/Indicative_Sanctions_Guidance_April_2009.pdf_28443340.pdf (accessed 24 March, 2011).
11. *Bolam v. Friern Barnet HMC.* All ER 118; 1957.
12. *Bolitho v. City and Hackney HA.* All ER 771; 1997.
13. *Pearce v. United Bristol Healthcare NHS Trust.* 48 BMLR 118; 1998.
14. Hart HLA. *The Concept of Law* [Chap. IX]. Oxford, England: Oxford University Press; 1961.
15. Hart HLA. *Law, Liberty and Morality* [Chap. I]. Oxford: Oxford University Press; 1962.
16. Worthington R. *Ethical and policy considerations of cardiopulmonary resuscitation.* In: Loftus R, editor. *Out-of-hours GP Toolkit.* London: Macmillan Cancer Support; 2008.

17. Murphy JB. *The Philosophy of Positive Law*. New Haven, CT: Yale University Press; 2005.
18. Coleman J, editor. *Hart's Postscript*. Oxford: Oxford University Press; 2001.
19. Coleman J. *The Practice of Principle: in defence of a pragmatist approach to legal theory* [Chap. VIII]. Oxford: Oxford University Press; 2001.
20. Rawls JA. *Theory of Justice*. Boston, MA: Harvard University Press; 1999.
21. NHS Litigation Authority Factsheet 2. Available at: www.nhsla.com/claims (accessed August 14, 2009).
22. Parliamentary and Health Service Ombudsman. *Remedy in the NHS: summary of recent cases*. London: PHSO; 2008: 21–22. Available at: www.ombudsman.org.uk/improving-public-service/reports-and-consultations/reports/health/remedy-in-the-nhs (accessed March 25, 2011).
23. Parliamentary and Health Service Ombudsman. *Principles for Remedy*. London: PHSO; 2009: 5. Available at: http://www.ombudsman.org.uk/improving-public-service/ombudsmansprinciples/principles-for-remedy (accessed April 22, 2011).

CHAPTER 3

Health policy and rationing: in search of reason

SOME BACKGROUND

Fresh attempts ought to be made to try and find a coherent rationale to deal with complex ethical issues in allocating resources for health care. It is known that resources are finite and that demand for health services is difficult to constrain; add to this increasingly expensive new medical technologies and it could be argued that problems associated with health care rationing can only get worse. This outlook is pessimistic, but there is often a reluctance to address problems of rationing head-on. The "R" word has strong political overtones, and frequent attempts are made to run away from it, and/or to pretend that it does not exist. Three R's—rationing, reality and reason—rarely co-exist, which ought not to be the case.

It is well known that cost, quality and access compete with one another when it comes to making decisions about prioritisation, and there is no simple formula that allows all three to flourish at the same time, enabling one to escape the so-called "iron triangle." By this it is meant that if quality is the main issue alongside access then costs tend to be a problem; if quality is the main concern along with affordability then access tends to suffer, and if costs are contained and access is given priority then a reduction in quality of services is a likely outcome. Given the no-win nature of this situation it is worth considering some theoretical frameworks as we believe there are more effective ways of dealing with these tensions.

FRAMEWORKS

Most people recognize that health care services are a finite resource and that there has to be an element of rationing and priority setting in the way that decisions are made about accessing treatment and allocating health care budgets. One framework that is widely used within this context is the QALY, or Quality Adjusted Life Year, which trades off the value of enjoying a healthy life against that of a less-healthy life measured in units of cost and time (*see* Chapter 4, page 44). While

QALYs are commonly employed as a policy tool they invariably mean: a) putting a monetary cost on a span of human life, and b) valuing one person's life higher than that of another by reason of that person having a disability or significant deficit in terms of his or her general health. This formula is discriminatory and it is open to question as to whether or not it has a legitimate basis for use within the context of *ethical* policy decision-making.

We propose that a more ethically appropriate and viable framework for those making policy decisions about rationing would follow these steps:

1 *Establish the nature of the task at hand*—Collate all the available evidence relating to: a) the needs of the patient or patient group in question; b) special circumstances (if any) that pertain to the case, including but not limited to scientific evidence; c) available resources needed to implement the change or offer the treatment over time, including human, financial and material costs; and d) relevant local and national guidelines set against any requirements in law.

2 *Directly consider the ethical dimension of the decision that needs to be made*—Refer to the available information, and a) see who stands to derive what benefit over what period of time and at what cost; b) identify any relevant and/or significant risks that might influence any decisions, and c) identify any burdens that could result in a negative impact being experienced by the patient.

3 *Establish what harms (if any) might be caused to others as a consequence of implementing a decision*—Consider the potential impact on others, including the community as a whole in clinical, social and economic terms, by asking whether funding one kind of treatment will lead to another one being withdrawn, restricted or downgraded in terms of prioritisation.

4 *Check for assumptions that are being made*—Consider possible alternatives that exist to the preferred course of action and be aware of any influences that might be being brought to bear on a decision; if no consensus is reached, then look for additional information or support and/or commission appropriate outside expertise, while at the same time applying the "mother test"—*how would you feel if it was your mother who was having restrictions placed on her in terms of accessing medical care?*

5 *Consider whether any aspects of a policy decision may eventually be subjected to legal challenge*—Consider the moral and legal basis of a decision (when made) to see if it stands up to close scrutiny, while remembering to keep accurate records and to communicate decisions to those who need to know.

This step-by-step approach should assist both clinicians and managers to make decisions about individual cases and help policy-setting, addressing primary areas of ethical and legal concern. The framework has the merit of asking the right questions in a simple, direct, ordered and coherent way, while at the same time considering important issues from different angles.

PUBLIC EXPECTATIONS

Part of the problem is that public expectations are often unrealistic in terms of the levels of care that can be afforded, for example, by the NHS. These expectations can nonetheless impact on policy-makers by exerting pressure to try and satisfy public demand for the provision of services. When the NHS was founded over 60 years ago medicine was a very different enterprise, and while the NHS has clear remnants of its original legacy in boasting universal access free at the point of need,[1] it is now trying to be more efficient in the name of modernization, and to be more consumer oriented in promoting patient choice while still trying to raise standards of care. All this presents a slightly impossible mix, since no health care system in the world can be all things to all people all of the time.

Society eventually has to make choices: how much health care does it want at what cost, and to whom should it be made available? Finding this balance has perhaps never been more difficult, but stumbling from crisis to crisis does nothing to help provide a coherent rationale for making change. Someone has to expend the effort and invest intellectual capital *before* deciding which way a new policy is going to lean.

What is certain is that because no single policy can point in two different directions, some form of policy equilibrium has to be established, neither pointing too far in one direction or the other. For instance, if the rights of individuals are considered to be of overriding importance, then it becomes a matter of logical necessity for public utility to suffer in some way. A problem that the NHS has at present is that the popularity that it enjoys from staying true to principles of open access is being challenged by a modernizing agenda prefaced on advocating greater patient choice. Of necessity, that is going to favour the individual over the interests of the community as a whole, thereby creating policy tension and some confusion of purpose.

If the NHS is going to reinvent itself, then it should not pretend to be one thing if in reality it is striving to be something else. Patients in the NHS cannot realistically have free and open choice to all the treatments they want, when they want it and at a facility of their choosing without constraints, all paid for out of central taxation. It would be a fiction to try and pretend that all this is achievable within the available resources. Such a level of service is normally the preserve of private medicine, and in terms of price, affordability and public policy, this level of choice can only be achieved by restricting access. The NHS cannot provide a whole range of alternatives while at the same time offering a universal service; therefore, in policy terms, it is disingenuous of any government to pretend that it can achieve all of these policy goals at once.

As a method of distribution, utility emphasizes "ends" at the expense of "means," which can be problematic when sacrifices need to be made along the way, such as causing one group of patients harm in order to benefit another, usually larger group of patients. The needs of the smaller group, for instance, could be pressing in kind even if few in number, and utility offers no ready solution for this kind of trade-off.[2]

There is value, however, in a system of wide distribution of essential goods and services such as health care, and utility should not just be dismissed out of hand. If universal access is the ultimate goal it can perhaps be achieved through genuine acceptance of a need to set limits, and focusing explicitly on the moral question of *how* this ought to be done. If rationing of services is not systematically approached, then patients may have to do without treatment, wait for long periods of time to receive treatment, or bypass the state system of provision—any or all of which could happen under the NHS. Use of co-payments where patients make a direct contribution towards the cost of an intervention is not a model that is currently used much in the UK. However, it has the merit of helping to achieve a fair, equitable distribution of risk and cost, and it would be surprising if this did not eventually become part of the process in distributing resources within the NHS.

TRANSPARENCY

Something that commonly arises in the context of decision-making when it comes to rationing is lack of transparency, and in practice it is often unclear who is making policy choices according to what criteria. While transparency in decision-making is sometimes debated,[3] an appropriate level of openness and public engagement is not the "norm," and neither is it always thought to be desirable. Nobody wants to be the one having to deny medical care to somebody else, whatever reasoning is applied. Similarly, not every doctor or care provider wants to be burdened by having to make difficult choices, and the line of least resistance is usually to leave it for someone else to make that decision. If decisions are often made at arm's length, it is ethically appropriate to consider which criteria are employed in making heath policy rationing decisions, both now and in the future.

It is impossible for every interested party to be involved in every rationing decision, but an ethical policy should attempt to involve those most affected by the outcome of a decision—in other words, *patients*. In the policy-making arena, lay (patient) representation is necessary though not sufficient, and on account of the number of factors that need to be taken into consideration when decisions are being made, then different types of expertise ought to be employed. Patients and professionals (or their representatives) as well as managers need to have their say, including politicians who are "running" the system. The real trick is trying to balance these different standpoints whilst actively addressing practical and economic necessities, all of this in the context of previous pre-existing policy objectives, which is clearly a tough challenge.

One cannot ignore the fact that these are ultimately political decisions, especially in the UK, where the Secretary of State for Health has the power to bring about significant change under delegated authority from Parliament. Doctors might resent what they see as undue interference by politicians, but this overlooks necessary social dimensions of medical practice. Medicine does not exist by and for itself. It exists (or ought to exist) to serve society, and in a democratic society it is politicians who are broadly speaking entrusted to make choices on behalf of others. Even if doctors do not directly engage in the process, they should acknowledge that their own decisions might have implications, such as how many patients they refer for tests, or how many prescriptions for medications they write as compared to the doctor up the street. That health care and politics co-exist is a given; *how* they interact is where ethics plays a part, and it is this dimension that needs further examination.

Ethical policies have to encompass all elements in the process of making decisions to provide, deny or restrict certain treatments. While these necessarily include politics and economics, incentives that reward doctors for being diligent gatekeepers of services can exert pressures of their own, and doctors are going to be influenced by financial incentives just the same as anybody else. Above all, ethical policies must be workable and applicable, with the ultimate aim of bringing benefit to the end-user, for which theory and practice need to work together.

We argue that key rationing criteria ought to include:

- the medical needs of patients
- the physical availability of resources relative to the needs of patients (including a patient's ability or inability to travel)
- fiscal arrangements for the provision of services, including the availability of specialist human resources and the need to work within budgetary constraints
- the cost of treatment and the length of time for which health care provision is likely to be needed
- the benefits, burdens and harms associated with treatment, relative to the needs of patients and the risks attached to receiving (or not receiving) treatment
- whether others are going to be disadvantaged as a result of providing a particular service, i.e. if the consequence is that resources are diverted away from one category of patient and on to another.

These six criteria sit alongside the five-stage framework described above, and they cover a spectrum of ideas including the needs and preferences of the individual, the needs of the health care professional, as well as the needs of the community as a whole.

POLICY FAILURE

Policies that lack flexibility are especially susceptible to failure; for example, policies that are too inclusive in terms of the range of services available could be harmful simply by placing an unreasonable burden on society as a whole. Policies that are too restrictive can also harm patients, and a society that is unable to care for those of its members who are unable to care for themselves is going to be morally difficult to defend. Patients sometimes suffer harms, up to and including death, if necessary treatment is withheld. This begs the question of what is meant by necessity; but that remains a separate issue. An ethical policy has to try and balance competing interests: the interests of society, the interests of the community and the interests of the individual. However, much of this combination may be elusive: if one factor becomes too dominant, then ways to minimize damage caused to other less-dominant factors will need to be explored.

Various devices exist for deferring difficult decisions on to someone else, and one method is for local providers to defer to national guidelines for help in determining what can and cannot be offered to particular patients. The validity of ethical criteria employed depends on how the deferral process works, and on the reliability and availability of good quality guidance. Deferral of decision-making is not unusual and is in many ways an everyday occurrence. It can work in both directions—away from government on to local clinical managers, or in the opposite direction and on to a body that is detached from decision-making about individual episodes of care.

Complex avoidance tactics are used by either side as a way of trying to avoid making explicit, hard choices. Neither doctors nor managers want to say: "Sorry, but I think your case is not sufficiently deserving, so I'm going to prioritize somebody else, and you will have to wait or make do without or with another less effective treatment" (this would be failing the "mother test," whereby something is acceptable for the public at large, but not for someone dear to you as an individual). In summary, we hold that anyone who has been adversely affected by a rationing decision has a moral right to know how that decision was made and to achieve what end.

NATIONAL VERSUS REGIONAL OR LOCAL

There is another confounding factor that needs to be addressed. For example, in the NHS, tensions exist between trying to meet centrally set targets while demonstrating respect for local decision-making that is based on trying to meet local needs. There is inevitability in terms of the ebb and flow between: determination of and compliance with locally-set objectives, and meeting targets set at a national level—often coercively. In the UK this situation is made more complex by a devolution agenda, with England, Wales, Scotland and Northern Ireland each having slightly different powers and responsibilities towards the provision of health services, e.g. Scotland has a devolved parliament and an entirely separate NHS.

This situation does not lead to an easy way of making and implementing coherent policy decisions about health, and in debating health policy the devolution effect must be acknowledged because of these additional and sometimes contradictory pressures. Health care providers such as hospitals and trusts may work with increasing levels of autonomy in terms of setting budgets and being responsible for local decisions on spending, but this must be viewed against a background where there remains a high-level, central government control.

Another confounding factor has to do with criteria employed for evaluating different types of treatment and the extent to which local choices are made. National decision-making can fail to take account of local population needs, and while this is the reasoning behind devolution, it cannot necessarily deliver on local agenda if decisions are still subject to control from central government. Rationing policy should be able to accommodate local needs without ignoring agenda set at the "higher" level, and the trick remains one of finding balance between competing pressures and priorities and finding a pathway through a maze of policies that are subject to change and internal contradiction. Individual practicing doctors, whether within the community or working in hospitals, are very much influenced by the situations described, even if they are content *not* to be part of the decision-making process.

EQUITY AND CLINICAL JUDGMENT

From an ethical perspective, it is difficult to ensure fairness and equity in terms of accessing treatment; this is an elusive goal, and the NHS is probably no nearer to achieving this now that it was 10 or even 20 years ago. Equity is not synonymous with *equality*—this would make the assumption that conditions of "health equality" are possible and achievable, but the need to achieve general conditions of equity in decision-making matters ought to feature more in the process of policy formulation.

Doctors have a part to play in terms of how individual clinical decisions are made, and their clinical judgment should not be subject to unreasonable challenge. Each decision doctors make to refer a patient on for specialist services or to write a prescription for a new expensive drug is influenced by or has some kind of influence on the system as a whole. Furthermore, if a treatment exists but cannot be offered to a particular patient because of cost constraints, it is fair to ask whether that patient ought to know that a treatment has been withheld. Patients' needs are paramount to the whole endeavour of providing health services; that should be stating the obvious but it is not always the case, and sick patients are never in a good position to defend their rights. Denying patients a form of care is one thing; denying them the right to know that they have been denied a treatment is morally harder to defend, even though not all patients would want to be burdened with such information or with having to make a choice.

NICE ROLES

Back in 1999, the Secretary of State for Health (England and Wales) acknowledged the need for equity, saying: "We want to tackle the unacceptable variations of service across the country, assuring quality and improving equity of access."[4] This remark prefaced the formation of the National Institute for Clinical Excellence (NICE), which is now the National Institute for Health and Clinical Excellence. This body was once referred to a little optimistically as one "of Britain's greatest cultural exports,"[5] but the organization has some policy contradictions of its own.

From the outset, its primary role was to review the evidence base and assess the clinical and cost effectiveness of new drugs and medical technologies. A secondary role, linked to the first, had to do with addressing variations in access to certain treatments and some of the growing disparities between people living in different postal areas. This kind of disparity runs contrary to the ethic of a *national* health service, but to judge from the evidence, variations between different post code areas appear to be worse—not better—than they were when NICE was set up,[6] and one has to ask "why." NICE makes *central* recommendations but they have to be implemented and resourced at local level, usually without matching funds, and this is perhaps why conditions of equity are becoming harder to attain, rather than easier.

Consider the following:

1 *Government wants to reduce variations between post code areas and reduce inequalities that exist in the provision of health services [p].*
2 *NICE is set up to assess the clinical and cost-effectiveness of new medical technologies, to produce guidance and to help address p [q].*

So far so good, but the connection between *p* and *q* has for unknown reasons neither been explained, proven nor seriously challenged.

Reducing health inequalities is a laudable goal, but as a concept, health *equality* may never be a reality, and if there is no established connection between *p* and *q* this presents a serious difficulty in terms of an organization being able meet its prime objectives.

If service providers pay attention to guidelines produced by NICE they can be forced to make the kinds of choices whereby funding one type of treatment means withholding or withdrawing funding for another, which gives rise to a certain circularity. Resources are always finite, and there is a certain inescapable logic that sees how new treatments and technologies being added by NICE puts pressure on budgets that cannot be stretched indefinitely, even with savings and efficiencies. A strong rationale for rationing is needed now even more than before. NICE does not *overtly* ration care but it clearly has a role to play in limiting access to expensive new treatments. If appraisals yield positive results, usually there is no dedicated trail of funding that follows in the wake of its recommendations. If implementing NICE guidance leads to a restriction in the provision of other services, the end result is still rationing and a reduction in equity between different categories of health services. Acknowledging this problem, NICE has now introduced policies on implementation,[7] even if it may never live up to the ideal and be able to reduce inequalities in health outcomes.

THE INFLUENCE OF COMMON LAW

In order to put the criteria into perspective it is worth considering rationing in relation to common law. That rationing happens is a matter of fact, not opinion, but *how* it happens is what gives rise to ethical concerns. A landmark English case settled on appeal in 2006 raises some interesting points. We are referring to Rogers v. Swindon,[8] a case which raised some interesting questions, namely:

- how much reliance should be placed on whether or not a drug is approved by NICE before decisions are made about local deliberations on whether or not a drug should be funded?
- to what extent should risk factors feature in decision-making about the appropriateness of a particular treatment (given that risk is always a factor in decision-making, whether at a public level or private)?
- what makes a case exceptional in terms of deviating from a generalized rule or set of principles?
- to what extent is cost the main issue when deciding whether or not a particular treatment should be funded?

During processes of deliberation about which group of patients should have access to which category of drug, the court made it clear that interim policies should be logical and internally consistent. If the processes of deliberation take a long time to complete, patients could be dying in the meantime from not having access to a treatment that would otherwise be available. This represents a particular form of moral hazard, and one that should be avoided.

In Rogers v. Swindon, a decision by the lower court not to fund a treatment was deemed to be "irrational and therefore unlawful,"[9] which led to the original adjudication being overturned. This appeal to logical reasoning means that in the future when making ethical judgments about resource-allocation, service providers must be able to defend the policy aspects of their reasoning. Therefore, logical and coherent policy decisions on rationing need to be based on general principles and rational argument, especially in deciding if, how and why to deviate from published guidelines.

NICE guidelines had been drawn up for the drug Herceptin® (*trastuzumab*) but not for a particular category of patient, namely early as opposed to late-stage breast cancer. While there was also a measure of clinical uncertainty about safety and efficacy, the patient did meet clinical and genetic criteria of eligibility for the treatment. This landmark ruling helped establish legal principles for making rationing decisions in the context of the NHS, the ethical nature of which have implications, whereby implementing guidance on a piecemeal basis with insufficient rational justification is now deemed unlawful. This case exposed the pitfalls in applying NICE guidelines, showing that on their own, the guidelines do not provide sufficient or appropriate mechanisms for making policy determinations about rationing.

A DIFFERENT APPROACH TO RATIONING

In the USA, the now famous Oregon Health Plan that began in the 1990s was an experiment to widen access to essential health care services, and was achieved by restricting access to treatments seen as being low priority. The relative importance of different types of treatment was determined locally, which in part happened by consulting public opinion. This was without precedent, and it should be seen against a background of a move towards the state-wide provision of universal health coverage, which remains a major topic of public debate. The Oregon example of health policy planning illustrates how different types of measures can be devised to try and address fundamental problems associated with trying to balance cost, quality and access. It has not been widely adopted but neither has it been abandoned. The objective in Oregon was to widen access for patients receiving state benefits, and not to cut costs.[10] What the Oregon planners did achieve was to use a policy mechanism that was open and transparent in the course of trying to achieve a long-term goal. In principle, this was an ethically sound initiative; however, the Oregon Plan "paradoxically made it harder for politicians to ration medical care and easier to raise funds for the state's poor."[11] This dual if unintended result may have arisen on account of the level of openness associated with the formulation of a policy that attracted much critical media attention. It proved very difficult to ration care through using a list of "approved" treatments that explicitly defined medical care priorities. Patients needing treatments that were not on the list either had to fund it themselves, which was not a viable option because the policy was specifically aimed at those receiving benefits, or go without.

The Oregon Plan was a bold initiative, but because of the nature of the exercise and the fact that it was influenced by local political factors, according to Marmor *et al.*, it should not be seen as a transferable model for making decisions on the allocation of health care resources.[12] This example of policy in action actually provides a counter-argument to the case for greater transparency, and where the public knows about individuals who are being denied some sort of care, it can provoke a hostile, negative reaction, however good the original intentions may have been.

CONCLUSION

Overall, this leaves us with rational decision-making as something upheld as a legal requirement in the UK, while in Oregon in the USA, public and transparent decision-making about rationing policy yielded some unwanted consequences, such that sick people of limited means were denied potentially life-saving medical care. Therefore, in terms of outcome, neither policy approach may have resulted in much public good. What is needed instead is an effective policy on controlling access to expensive treatments that is equitable and follows broad principles that can be commonly applied, thus eliminating some of the worst discrepancies in terms of variations in access to different levels of care.

An ethical policy should be capable of adapting to local differences of administration and law, and it ought to recognize that different needs exist in relation to different categories of local service provision. It should be transparent in so far as patients and professionals should know where they stand. Finally, an ethical policy should help reduce the risk of policy contradiction and failure, which happens if and only if there is in an appropriate level of clarity in the process.

There may be no "right" way of dealing with rationing, but there are more ethical ways of doing it than those that all too often operate by default. Doctors and patients do not need to be policy experts, but they need to be able to question decisions, and to know who is making them for whose benefit, and according to what criteria. Such an approach towards the formulation of public policy should help to promote overall conditions of equity, the key ingredients being respect for principles of equity and transparency and principles of service provision aimed at maximizing benefit in terms of patient outcomes. This may sound like a wish list, but we believe that unless this difficult discussion is engaged in openly and directly, and unless goals are clear in terms of rationing policy objectives, then the end result is often ethically problematic and morally difficult to defend.

A HYPOTHETICAL CASE

It is worth constructing a hypothetical case to work through some of these principles in order to illustrate them further and enable a critical appraisal of frameworks outlined at the beginning of this chapter. A good example would be to explore possible trade-offs between providing funding for assisted reproduction as opposed to mental health services for the young. Both type of provision are likely to be required by a small but significant percentage of the population but for quite different reasons. Neither situation involves the provision of critical care, but both have significant implications for those affected. Couples unable to conceive on their own may not be in a position to afford private treatment, and young people suffering from depression, addiction and psychological disturbances may have nowhere else to go for help. Both situations, therefore, have equally bad consequences for those who are affected. Some categories of treatment, such as the ones we are describing, are seen as "soft targets," and assisted reproductive treatments and mental health services can both fall under this heading.

Cutting beds in an acute hospital, for instance, would be a much more visible thing to do, and as a result, much more damaging politically; therefore, emergency medicine is never seen as a soft target. Central government can make choices; however, local health service providers, such as clinics and hospitals, have to be able to offer a range of services based on priorities that have been agreed upon locally as well as on the availability of funding. The nature of the task is to find an ethical way of balancing the competing need for scarce resources.

Clinical and scientific evidence must be weighed up, and details of local needs must to be reviewed in the light of the evidence. Only at this point can available resources be allocated, making it clear how decisions were made while having respect for the law and for other policy previous commitments (to avoid having to take away something that was previously available). Benefits and costs must also be assessed in relation to long-term clinical and social needs and the likely outcomes of a decision, i.e. not just in relation to immediate financial or political objectives. Other people may be affected by this policy decision besides those who are in direct need of health services.

A complicating factor in our hypothetical case is that mental health patients can pose an immediate threat to themselves and/or to the safety of others in the community, whereas risks to individual couples in terms of reproductive choice is more of a private matter. This means that one is not comparing like with like, and trying to trade off such different health needs is not entirely logical. Nonetheless, a huge organization such as the British NHS provides a wide range of health services, and because budgets have to be balanced, trading off different categories of treatment such as assisted reproductive treatments and mental health services must sometimes be done.

When making rationing policy decision, relative harms need to be weighed against known risks, and who stands to benefit and to what extent from which course of action. The couple who might not be able to afford the private treatment needed in order to help them conceive will suffer in terms of quality of life and being unable to fulfill their own personal goals, whereas the outlook for the young mental health patient, who could have a treatable condition, is generally rather bleak. His entire life could be blighted if he is denied treatment when it is needed; he could become suicidal, or he could have a lifetime of suffering from depression, none of which are simply "fixed" by spending cash later.

One feature these two types of patient have in common is having limited opportunities to be able to achieve their respective life goals, with the possibility that a refusal of funding for treatment is denying these patients hope for the future. But if a choice has to be made, then in this instance, the young man with the mental needs would probably take priority because of his profile and because of risk-benefit ratios associated with treatment as opposed to non-treatment in his case. The couple wanting to start a family could argue that their human rights have been infringed, but that argument necessarily means that somebody else is obligated to provide the means of fulfilling those needs, which would be a very difficult position to defend.

Ethical, pragmatic rationing may not be easy but it ought not to be impossible, and it is hoped that some of the ideas explored in this chapter should have practical applications when applied in "real life."

REFERENCES

1. Rivett GC. *National health service history.* Available at: www.nhshistory.net (accessed August 20, 2009).
2. Smart JJC, Williams B. *Utilitarianism: For and Against.* Cambridge: Cambridge University Press; 1973.
3. *Rationing and the NHS* [symposium report]. *Drug Ther Bull.* 2003; **41**(7): 55–6.
4. Department of Health. *National standards will ensure equality of patient care.* Previously available at: www.dh.gov.uk/en/Publicationsandstatistics/Pressreleases/DH_4025357 (accessed August 20, 2009).
5. Smith R. The triumph of NICE. *B Med J.* 2004; **329**.
6. White C. *NICE guidance has failed to end 'postcode prescribing'. Brit Med. J.* 2004; **328**: 1277.
7. National Institute for Health and Clinical Excellence. *Putting NICE guidance into practice.* NICE Implementation program, London, September 2009. Available at: www.nice.org.uk/media/E7B/C4/PuttingNICEGuidanceIntoPractice2009.pdf (accessed March 25, 2011).
8. *Rogers v. Swindon.* EWCA Civ 392; 2006. Available at: www.bailii.org/cgi-bin/markup.cgi?doc=/ew/cases/EWCA/Civ/2006/392.html&query=title+(+rogers+)+and+title+(+v+)+and+title+(+swindon+)&method=boolean (accessed September 8, 2009).
9. Ibid.
10. Jacobs L, Oblander J, Marmor T. The Oregon Health Plan and the political paradox of rationing. *J Health Politics, Policy and Law.* 1999; **24**(1): 161–80.
11. Marmor T. *Lessons from Oregon.* In: Hackey R, Rochefort D, editors. *The New Politics of State Health Policy.* Kansas, USA: University of Kansas Press; 2001.
12. Ibid.

CHAPTER 4

Policy success and failure: causes, remedies and methods of analysis ·

Health policy is a fast-moving subject; however, when the Royal Society of Medicine put on an exhibition in London in 2008 to commemorate the British National Health Service's 60th anniversary, one could not help but notice that when comparing documents from 1968, 1988 or 2008 that some of the content was strikingly similar. While health policy records reveal much about a time and place, some themes keep recurring and problems sometimes never go away. Thus for the analyst there is a benefit to be gained from taking the long view.

When analyzing policy change it seems that new policies often fail to address the fundamentals and acknowledge the underlying nature of the problem being addressed. Health policy can as easily be plagued by poor design as by poor implementation, and organizational change in health care is sometimes akin to re-arranging office furniture without knowing either whether the old arrangement worked or what benefits the new arrangement is meant to bring. It is also often the case that benefits of policy change are over-stated, effectively meaning that the "old furniture" is still there even if it is in a different place. Therefore, if a previous policy was never evaluated or had not been in existence for long, then any new policy stands a high chance of failing to meet its objectives, however glamorous and innovative it might appear at the time. Change for change's sake never achieves much, and change driven by the need for short-term gain, whether political, financial or both, may have similar characteristics. Proposed change that does nothing to alter the nature of an enterprise is largely futile, which in a health care context essentially means failing to improve service provision for patients.

PATIENT CARE

Patient benefit is sometimes well down the list of priorities in cases where service "improvements" are aimed at the provider more than the user, in other words, at trying to ensure better outcomes and address patients' needs. If both these objectives coincide the result is positive all round; however, it is fair to question the *frequency* with which this happens, as well as to question the underlying *intentions* behind many changes in policy. Intention is pivotal in terms of understanding and predicting future policy success and failure, and it is worth examining critically *why* policies fail to meet their objectives and yield the anticipated results, and why if policies do work, success is not always properly attributed. For instance, have the right questions been asked, has an improvement been brought about by an effective policy intervention, or has it been brought about by something else, such as a trend already taking place?

While the broad contention behind this book is that incorporating *ethical* analysis into policy development offers a potential remedy for some of the causes of policy failure, there is no suggestion that merely factoring in ethics will provide a panacea. There is a suggestion, however, that policy that has been ethically evaluated ought to lead to greater effectiveness when put into action. This is from having taken into account the moral basis of an argument to pursue (or not to pursue) a particular course of action, and from having had the benefit of perspective into the nature of the problems being addressed.

Policy analysis may be an art, but it should still be scientific in its methods and thus should employ principles of logic as well as the analysis of statistics. In short, it is important to know the value of a thing and not just its price.[1] Analyzing the cost of health care in the same way as analyzing the cost of a tin of beans or a gallon of fuel can lead to perverse results because the nature of health care is so different from other more tangible commodities. The most sophisticated analysis of the cost of providing a clinical episode of care, for instance that of a hip replacement, does nothing in terms of measuring the cost to an individual of a procedure that is delayed, or one that goes wrong or one that cannot be given at all. Neither can it accurately measure the impact on society in terms of patient wellbeing, or patients' ability to function as full, active members of their community.

POLICY CONTRADICTIONS

Normal rules of logic dictate that if a policy is based on all false premises it cannot succeed in meeting its objectives because the conclusion of such an argument will also be false. Similarly, if two policies are pointing in opposite directions at the same time, the list of possible outcomes is short. Either one policy fails or they both fail, because push-pull policies invariably cancel each other out. It cannot be the case that each policy will have a limited measure of success when success in one area comes at the direct expense of another. In that situation, neither policy will succeed in meeting its primary objectives and money and effort will have been spent in the process to no avail.

One such policy contradiction comes about when political attempts at *de-*centralization clash with measures requiring uniform standards and thus for government control to be strengthened, e.g. causing locally set budgets to be spent according to agendas set by central government. One requires good local governance and levels of accountability; the other requires strong government and for compliance to be demonstrated by local officials. To take an example, directives intended to drive down infection rates for one type of hospital-acquired infection could be at odds with local level executive decisions aimed at reducing *all* types of infection. Where this happens, policies originating from the center are the ones that usually dominate, because central government has the power to impose policy, meaning that local initiatives are usually the ones that end up having to be dropped.

Central "command and control" tactics have long been part of the day-to-day operation of the NHS, which some people view as a strength and others as a weakness. In a time of cutbacks and reform this centralized structure can offer significant advantages, but it can also lead to conflict between central government's wishes and policy decisions that are best agreed locally. Tensions always exist between central and local government; this kind of tension invariably affects the way in which policies are developed and implemented, wherever the balance of power lies. It should always be clear who is responsible when policy changes the way that health care is provided; the way in which local health management structures are organized and run is as important as the role played by central government.

PUBLIC VERSUS PRIVATE

In late 2008 a policy initiative announced by the British Government went to the heart of the British National Health Service when a report commissioned by the Secretary of State for Health on improving access to medicines for NHS cancer patients was released.[2] It focused on the high cost of new generation drugs for treating cancer and the fact that hospitals and trusts were not always prepared to meet the cost. The key feature of the new policy is that patients can receive the rest of their treatment through the NHS, no longer having to choose between two extremes by: a) having all private medical treatment or b) something fully funded by the state. The basic premise upon which the NHS was founded was to provide access to health care that what was free at the point of need, irrespective of patients' ability to pay. For 60 years patients either elected to go outside the system and receive treatment as a private patient or to be treated exclusively within the NHS. Previously the NHS did not permit top-ups or contributions to be made by patients.

Implications for this policy change could lead to reduced levels of equity within the system if patients that can afford it pay for part of their treatment, but others that cannot afford to pay have to make do with older, less expensive or less effective treatments. Patients could decide to sell their homes to pay for the drugs that promise the potential to prolong life. But if the drug therapy lacks an evidence base or is considered too experimental in nature, then even if patients can afford it is it right to allow patients to take these risks for such an uncertain outcome? This new policy is short on logic because if there is strong evidence that a particular medicine works then it is quite likely to be available under the NHS.

This type of decision is usually made by NICE. Now it seems that the public must sometimes make decisions on its own, which may be democratic and support individual patient autonomy, but one has to ask whether patients are properly equipped to make such decisions, and what happens to equity within the system as a whole. Patients who have a terminal illness may have a choice of sorts, but the ethics of the policy do not seem to have been properly thought through.

Equity in the system as a whole is weakened when patients who can afford "better," more expensive drugs with better potential outcomes decide to meet the cost based on what their local service is able to provide and how much money they have in the bank. Such policies are standard practice in many countries but they are new within the NHS. Having in mind the discussion in Chapter 3 about the purpose of NICE, this further shows that it is unclear what a policy such as this is trying to achieve other than to pass costs for certain types of treatment on to patients and away from the NHS. This is rationing, not an exercise in promoting individual patient choice, and it is one that is based on an unclear social policy agenda and a doubtful application of ethics.

The boundaries between state and private health care are now more porous than they were, and NHS patients with cancer can be seen at a private hospital for treatment, or patients funded by a private insurer can be seen for part of their treatment at an NHS facility (especially a large teaching hospital with access to the latest modern technologies). It is no longer the case that all patients in one type of hospital are treated on the same basis. This blurring may not matter to some but it makes transparency harder to achieve, and the policy would fail the rationality test described in the previous chapter.

QALYs

If rationality is a criterion of legal validity in terms of the allocation of resources,[3] then the maximum figure of £30000 per annum that has been employed in the UK for making rationing-type decisions—based on the formula of a "cost per Quality Adjusted Life Year" (QALY)—seems somewhat arbitrary.[4] This formula works on the basis whereby:

> "a single QALY would indicate one year in perfect health. The value of a year in less than perfect health would be a fraction (e.g. 0.5) of a QALY. Improvements in length and quality of life are referred to as fractions of a QALY."[5]

The reasoning behind QALYs has other problems besides a doubtful basis in logic, in that as suggested in the last chapter, it discriminates between the value of a life lived in perfect health and one lived with disabilities. To a person with disabilities, life could have equal or greater value when measured against the values that such a person held prior to becoming disabled, and while it is easy to take being healthy for granted, it is unethical to assume that *not* being healthy is equivalent to being "*half*-alive." Reservations remain, therefore, about the ethical validity of using this as a policy tool, and in the case of drugs that we were discussing previously, is treatment under the NHS being refused on grounds of cost-per-QALY or on grounds of unproven efficacy? If the latter, this begs the question of how and why drugs are given a license. If it is about rationing, then that should be made clear.

THE VALUE OF INFORMATION

Policy obfuscation arises where there is a deliberate attempt to mislead, which can happen for example, with selective publication of "news" and by withholding information about policy contradictions when they are known about but ignored. These are not hypothetical situations, and from a policy perspective, lack of clarity presents real dangers when health is the subject under discussion. Disinformation can sometimes present a greater harm to patients than no information at all, and in terms of ethical criteria, members of the public, any and all of whom are would-be patients, have a right to know the reasoning behind any given policy.

One justification for making an exception to this general rule would be if publicly accessible information were to cause patients anxiety or alarm, which might in turn lead to a refusal to follow "expert" advice. But it can also work in the opposite direction and lead to risk-averse decision-making and to paternalistic decisions being made by central government. It is a matter of political as well as scientific judgment to decide how much information to place in the public domain and how much to attempt to withhold. But ethically it is usually better to trust patients than to withhold information that permits people to make informed decisions, unless the stakes really are too high in relation to the common good. There are few defensible reasons why the public cannot have the information that it needs in order to be able to reach a judgment.

POLICY CONTRADICTIONS (REVISITED)

Policy confusion arising from a contradiction that has been overlooked is less troubling from a moral perspective than something that is deliberately concealed, but contradictions should not happen if serious thought is given to what a policy is meant to achieve and how it should work *in practice*. Governments do not usually lack access to good advice, it being more likely to be the case that there is an abundance of advice available to civil servants and ministers, even if it does not all point in one direction. Therefore, there are no justifiable excuses for introducing policies that contradict one another, especially when public consultation is commonly built into the design phase of most policy development strategies.

Where government departments and regulatory agencies consult on new policy and guidance, it is respectful of human rights to allow interested parties to contribute to the process, and to be able to express opinions ahead of final decisions being made about the introduction of a new policy. However, for consultations to be effective they should be part of a coordinated approach of public engagement to prevent them from being exercises in public relations. This can include focus groups or face-to-face meetings with people likely to be affected by the implementation of any new policy. Public consultation improves transparency and accords with wider principles of democratic justice, even if the process is not always readily accessible to people outside the world of policy. It takes time to respond, and one has to know about a consultation in the first place.

This level of engagement has the potential to result in changes being made before a new policy is introduced. In the case of professional guidance for doctors, this could lead to changes to the guidance after a draft has been issued. Similarly, codes of practice laying out how new acts of parliament are intended to work could (or should) end up being amended after input from professionals and the public. (This happened in the case of the Mental Capacity Act (2005) that became effective in 2007 after a reasonably high level of public engagement; changes were thought necessary even though the final version of the Code of Practice relating to the Act did not meet everyone's expectations.)

Clearly, if half of all respondents hold one view and the other half an opposing view, then it has to be down to advisers and experts (or the minister in charge) to reach a decision on the best way forward. Nonetheless, policy has greater social validity for having been through the process and from having had the benefit of being openly discussed. This level of engagement not only permits open discourse but has the potential to prevent misunderstandings from arising, and preventing something deeply unpopular from being introduced. (This was the case with mental health reform in England; attempts by government to introduce new legislation culminated in 2007 in an amendment to an *old* Mental Health Act dating back to 1986, on account of widespread objections to a proposed new act that eventually had to be withdrawn.)[6]

If, after a process of pubic engagement, during the final stage of policy development a government minister decides to veto amendments arising from the process, this would not be unlawful in so far as ministers are invested with the authority to devise policies and to put them into action. But whether such conduct would be ethically acceptable is more of an open question. An inherent risk in policy development is the fact that sometimes ministers are no longer in office when a policy works through to the point where it is tested in action. In the case of the second half of a four-year term of government, the chances of a policy being evaluated and of the individual government minister responsible for a new policy still being in office are tiny. Holding consultations is no substitute for good policy formulation, and while policy confusion can still come about it is less likely to come about if a meaningful consultation has taken place.

If public bodies are serious about this and about implementing ideas that will work, then from an ethical perspective, time and energy should be spent in seeking well-informed opinions as well as looking for possible contradictions. This is only possible if policies that are already in place have been properly assessed, and in health care this rarely happens. For one thing, data collection is administratively complex and expensive, and for another, the process takes a long time, and because policies are often introduced in fairly rapid succession, there may be little or no opportunity for this type of evaluation to happen.

HUMAN ERROR AND QUESTIONS OF PROBITY

Human error presents its own challenges, and policies can fail because of something totally unforeseen. Policy probity is effectively the opposite of policy harm, and to take a practical example, an Australian policy of open disclosure emphasising probity (in all but name) has been introduced in New South Wales.[7] It encouraged clinicians to explain, apologize and reassure patients in cases where error had occurred. This kind of openness is not common in medicine and it will be interesting to see evaluation results once the policy has been in place for a few years. (A similar policy is finding its way over to Britain.)

The issue of unexplained medically induced deaths dramatically came to public attention in the UK in early 2009 when a government-sponsored commission published a report into unexplained deaths at hospitals in the West Midlands.[8] This caused shock to patients, professionals and managers alike, and not only at the hospitals in question. It led to local changes in senior management and to accusations being levelled against the government with regard to suggestions that deaths had come about as a consequence of central government policies that the hospitals felt compelled to implement.[9]

One of the issues in this case was about waiting times in the emergency department before a patient is assessed by a qualified person. This, it was decided, should be no more than four hours, but blanket policies based on the amount of time elapsing between a patient being brought in by ambulance and a patient being seen by a doctor take no account of different patients' medical needs, or of the fact that junior doctors often do the initial evaluation, and it can take a much longer time for a patient to be seen by a specialist. This kind of waiting is not taken into account according to central government criteria.

Patients can die through decisions having been made at government level in just the same way that patients can die through local systems errors, or through mistakes that are made by doctors, any and each of which are potentially dangerous. Where medical judgment is distorted by *bad* policy it can lead to preventable and significant harm being done to patients. When in the USA news of the Institute of Medicine's report *To Err is Human* came out in 1999, it broke a taboo by openly putting forward estimated statistics about medically induced deaths associated with human error.[10] Since that time, medical error and patient safety have moved higher up the political agenda, but there is always a sense of public shock when information comes to light about patients dying as a result of unintended consequences associated with failing or dysfunctional health systems, or trusted but fallible health care professionals. This is the sharp end of policy, where decisions made at a distance have direct implications, for example, affecting every emergency department in the country—hence the seriousness of this endeavour.

SUMMARY

For policies to be effective there ought to be clarity about what a policy change is meant to bring about or what policy failings are meant to be corrected. The policy-maker therefore needs to have clear goals as well as clarity about what is wrong with existing arrangements. It makes no sense to introduce new policy without allowing time for previous policies to be implemented and evaluated. Policies so easily fail at this stage, and this basic criterion of policy formulation and development is rarely met. Armed with clarity of purpose and good quality data—then and only then—should the real work of policy development and re-evaluation start.

The potential impact of any new policy must be considered, including how it meshes with other policies. Missing out on this step leaves open the possibility, if not the inevitability, that policy contradictions will militate against the new initiative. This stage is part of a process rather than a point in time, and it is essential that proper resources are allocated to the task. Before adoption and implementation, everyone affected by the introduction of new policy, such as patients groups, health care professionals, and voluntary sector bodies, should have the chance to be involved. Recognizing that special interest groups have their own agenda and that they may not always be objective in making comments and criticisms, checks and balances need to be incorporated into the process of engagement. When a final policy document is drafted, analysts can afford more or less weight to different opinions according to their relevance and to primary motivations and intentions behind the change. This stage is not about following rules; it is about critical evaluation, which requires both skill and clarity of thinking; it should not be rushed, and realistic deadlines ought to be set.

IMPLEMENTATION

Publication of a policy document or new piece of guidance is not the end of the matter, and if publication is no more than that then the process is not complete. Implementation is a crucial stage in policy development, and stakeholders need to know about a change as well be provided with background information about why it is being introduced. It should not be left to health professionals and others to find out about a new policy by chance and to then have to figure out what it means.

Help may be needed when it comes to putting policy into practice, and this will require resources to be committed to the process. The dissemination process is always partly educational, and if appropriate resources are not made available at this stage, the result could be another new policy having to be devised to fix a policy that merely *appears* not to be working. If anticipated results do not manifest themselves, then someone should be asking why. The right course of action might be simply to allow a policy time to 'bed in', or if necessary, to devise measures or interventions to fix any problems that have arisen. Good policy can easily fail because it is not properly implemented and assessed, and dissemination work must be carefully planned.

These different stages characterize the endeavour of policy formulation and development, and each is more or less interdependent with the other. If shortcuts are made and corners cut then policy failure is more likely, and new health policies should have these phases built in as a matter of course. This not only helps establish ethical validity for new policies but it makes it more likely that they will achieve their primary goal. Ethical validity depends on content as well as process, and it is not sufficient simply to ask, "Is there an ethical issue that needs to be considered?" by treating ethics as an afterthought or supplementary question (assuming ethics is considered at all). To ignore it is to miss out a crucial aspect of the process of policy development.

INTERNATIONAL COMPARATIVE POLICY ANALYSIS

The task of analyzing policy is more difficult when it is not confined to a single country or geographical region. Structures for health care delivery need to be broadly similar for direct comparisons to work, and even within the European Union (EU), for instance, this is not always the case. To take an example, public policy towards the provision of treatment for assisted conception varies in terms of both access and who pays for treatment between parts of the UK, to say nothing of the EU as a whole. Making broad comparisons requires an understanding of the health care delivery systems that operate in each country before being able to make sense of what the different policies mean in practice.

When comparing situations that differ in so many ways it is important to acknowledge this and to make allowances for any known confounding variables, i.e. factors that can derail the process. Marmor, Freeman and Okma rightly point out that this is no trivial task.[11] International policy comparison, regrettably, does not always take this into account and demonstrate appropriate levels of sophistication. One might read, for instance, about UK government officials looking to the USA to "see how things are done over there," as if health policy were a settled matter, ignoring the fact that health policy is fast changing, and is in case usually determined at state rather than federal level. Naivety and over-simplification are as much pitfalls to good policy-making as failing to take account of known, contradictory premises.

When Marmor notes differences between learning *about* policy processes in a country and learning *why* they are the way they are, essentially he is pointing to differences between observation and analysis.[12] One precedes the other, and one without the other is not a good harbinger of change. Even august public international bodies are not infallible when it comes to pitfalls in comparative policy analysis, and the World Health Organization *2000 World Health Report* was roundly criticised for methodological error.[13,14] In order to make observations that have meaning and relevance it is important to consider the social background to each individual policy that is applicable to any given country. This is in addition to paying attention to dominant economic and political factors that can affect how policies work. False comparisons only mislead, and when such information ends up in the public domain it can be quoted and re-quoted, thus compounding original errors.

International comparative analysis is multifaceted, and while Part 3 of this book comments on key features of the case studies in Part 2, the intention here is not to *devise* policy but to consider how it should be assessed, formulated and implemented. Comparisons made for the purpose of developing new policy need to be specific and detailed, and failing to take account of complexity not only misses the point but commits an ethical fallacy. Misinforming the public does no service to anyone, and in the domain of cross-country comparisons as well as in the domain of country specific policy analysis, moral considerations need to be an active part of the process of deliberation. Myths about "ethics-free zones" present just as much danger in international settings as they do when analyzing policy within a country.

Meaningful international comparative health policy analysis does not always receive the attention it deserves. What gives meaning to the process is depth of insight, which does not come from making comparisons that merely draw parallels or describe basic differences. Insights can be derived from good statistical analysis but they can also be derived from analyzing the moral elements of policy; for instance, by reflecting on the extent of certain health policy aspects addressing actual patient needs. This is not so much about making judgments about one system against another but about shared learning and collective experiences, asking "which system best serves the needs of patients and why." This is the real value of the exercise, and it is worth reminding ourselves that health care is ultimately about providing a service, whether for profit or as a matter of public utility. As such there will always be a moral dimension, whether or not it is formally acknowledged.

REFERENCES

1. Ackerman F, Heinzerling L. *Priceless: on knowing the price of everything and the value of nothing.* New York, NY: The New Press; 2004.
2. Richards M. *Improving access to medicine for NHS patients.* London: The Stationary Office; 2008.
3. *See* Chapter 3.
4. House of Commons Health Committee First Report of Session 2007–8 (HC 27-I). *National Institute for Health and Clinical Excellence, Volume 1.* London: The Stationary Office; 2008. Available at: www.publications.parliament.uk/pa/cm200708/cmselect/cmhealth/27/27.pdf (accessed July 21, 2009).
5. Ibid.
6. *The blight and proper treatment of mental illness. The Times* [online]. May 16, 2007. Available at: www.timesonline.co.uk/tol/comment/letters/article1795574.ece (accessed July 19, 2009).
7. New South Wales Department of Safety and Quality Branch: Policies and procedures for open disclosure. *State-wide Implementation of Open Disclosure: Because it's the right thing to do.* Sydney, Australia; 2008. Available at: www.health.nsw.gov.au/resources/quality/opendisc/pdf/swide_implementation.pdf (accessed July 20, 2009).
8. Healthcare Commission. *Investigation into Mid Staffordshire NHS Foundation Trust* [report]. London: Healthcare Commission; 2009. Available at: http://image.guardian.co.uk/sys-files/Guardian/documents/2009/03/17/Investigation_into_Mid_Staffordshire_NHS_Foundation_Trust_Summary.pdf (accessed July 18, 2009).
9. *NHS targets 'may have led to 1,200 deaths in Mid-Staffordshire'. The Telegraph.* March 18, 2009. Available at: www.telegraph.co.uk/health/healthnews/5008935/NHS-targets-may-have-led-to-1200-deaths-in-Mid-Staffordshire.html (accessed July 18, 2009).
10. Institute of Medicine. *To Err is Human: building a safer health system.* Washington, DC: IOM; 1999. Available at: www.iom.edu/CMS/8089/5575.aspx (accessed December 28, 2008).
11. Marmor T, Freeman R, Okma K. *Comparative Perspectives and Policy: learning in the world of health care. J of Comparative Policy Analysis.* 2005; 7(4): 331–48.
12. Ibid. Sub-section: Summary and conclusion.
13. World Health Organization. *World Health 2000.* Geneva: WHO; 2000.
14. Williams A. A commentary on world health. *Health Economics.* 2000; **10**(2): 93–100.

PART 2

CHAPTER 5

Ancient origins and modern approaches to health care delivery in China

a) Medical ethics, policy and health care delivery in modern China

Kwok-Yin Chan

INTRODUCTION

Western accounts of medical ethics, originating from the time of Hippocrates, are not the only ones in existence today, and alternative systems of medicine, particularly originating in the East, have developed their own individual forms of medical ethics. Traditional Chinese medicine practiced over several millennia has its own underpinning ethical values, and these were profoundly influenced by Chinese culture and by Confucianism. Although Chinese medical theories are broadly irreconcilable with modern Western medicine, Chinese medical ethics shares certain commonalities as well as some unique concepts that merit serious consideration.

Medical practitioners in China have enjoyed high social status since the Song Dynasty (960–1279 AD). They are stereotypically academics and "bearers of impeccable moral values and conduct," and they are expected to exemplify and conform to the teachings of Confucianism. Western medical influence in China began in the 19th century, and traditional Chinese medicine (in terms of theory and technical advancement) was greatly influenced by the introduction of Western empirically based systems of medical knowledge. Modern scientific theories have gradually been replacing abstract traditional theories, such as Yin and Yang and the five-element theories, within mainstream medical practice.

Although Western medicine has been the dominant medical system in practice for the past century, medical ethics in China retained influences from the traditional Confucian-based system of medical practice. This phenomenon is largely attributed to cultural compatibility and to the systems of social values that currently exist in China. However, current inequalities within the Chinese health care system, in terms of access and distribution of resources in the wake of recent economic reforms, challenge some aspects of Western medical ethics. The aim of this chapter is to explore the characteristics of modern medical ethics in China and to see how this affects state policy and the methods of health care delivery.

CHINESE MEDICAL ETHICS

Chinese medical ethics derives its fundamental principles from Confucianism. According to the "Analects of Confucius" the standard of morality is summarised by using one word: "仁" (ren). This Chinese word is a combination of two different words that mean "thousand hearts." No English terminology can sufficiently convey this meaning, but one may interpret the word as a combination of the concepts of respect, benevolence, compassion, faithfulness, cooperation, sympathy and sensitivity. These virtues have influenced every facet of the Chinese society, and they are unparalleled by any other school of thought. They have long been considered part of the Chinese identity.

In Chinese terms, good medical practice is known as '仁术' (renshu), meaning "the art of benevolence," and this Confucian concept was further developed by famous physician Sun Simiao in the Tang Dynasty (618–907 AD).[1] Simiao is known for his writings on "the truth of sincerity in great physicians." These writings formally set the standard of medical ethics of ancient China, in a similar way that the Hippocratic Oath did in the West. Simiao's text instructs good physicians to be competent in their skills, to be wise and efficient in their practices, to be sincere to patients, to demonstrate goodwill, and to strive to ensure the preservation of life, which is of the utmost importance, as no other action is considered comparable. The text also gives emphasis to the importance of humility and humanity, and a physician should be unprejudiced with regard to the social class, wealth, age, political views and race of his patients. The ultimate aim is to build these virtues so as to influence physician behaviour to the extent of being able to limit and control personal values in doctors' clinical practice, minimizing bias and potential prejudice for the greater good of patients and others.

However, it is interesting that when Western and Chinese medical ethics are closely compared, the basic constructs have certain similarities. For instance, "doctors should do no harm" and must "always act in the best interest of the patient", although in practice there is a difference of approach towards patients and the decision-making process. In the West, medical professionals focus on the attainment of professional standards, and they are required to conduct themselves appropriately and to function within certain limits. A lesser emphasis is placed on individual moral aspirations, just as long as recognized standards have been met. On the other hand, Chinese medical professionals place greater focus on inner ethical qualities, and doctors should consistently reflect on whether their professional and personal behaviours conform to the ideology of the Confucian "art of benevolence." Traditional Chinese medicine practitioners believed that by conducting themselves in this fashion their practice would be safe and of a high standard, and that they would be less likely to be in breach of the law. There are no external, independent professional bodies that govern professional standards, as these are monitored and policed by the state.

One may argue that from an ethical standpoint the true question is whether the desire for ethical practice is coming from within or guided from without. This difference of internal "regulation" versus external regulation is a key point of different between Chinese and Western approaches to medical ethics. In some countries, such as the UK, medical ethics leans towards utilitarianism, which stipulates that for actions to be moral they should yield the maximum benefit overall.[2] This symbolizes a difference in approach, because whereas the East focuses more on virtues and character and whether primary intentions are genuinely noble, the Western utilitarian approach places greater emphasis on the consequences of a given course of action. However, this is not the only Western ethical construct, and in some respects the Kantian ethic of placing emphasis on the quality of an act rather than its consequences resembles Confucian ideals as an embodiment of the ethics of virtue. In contemporary Western philosophy, virtue ethics is sometimes even seen as being a separate branch of ethics.[3]

ECONOMIC REFORM, MEDICAL ETHICS AND HEALTH CARE DELIVERY

In recent years the practice of both traditional and Western medicine in China has become more receptive to the mode of Western medical ethics. This is in part due to globalization,[4] and in part due to the rapid economic development that has led to unprecedented demands for health care services.

The use of Western medicine has now become the dominant medical system in practice, and its evidence-based practice and effectiveness in reducing the mortality and morbidity over a spectrum of diseases is recognized by the public. Although being far more expensive, Western medicine remains the system of choice with exceptions due to personal choice and preferences. Therefore, the application of Western medical ethics and ideals of professionalism are in some ways a logical choice for maintaining standards of service and care.

Chinese economic reforms that began in 1978 have transformed economic structures away from a socialist-planned economy and towards a more market-based economy. The health care system has yet to achieve long-term sustainable conditions from a financial, structural and policy point of view, and while China may have the fastest growing national economy in the world,[5] this has resulted in a significant change in living standards between urban and rural populations. This in turn translates into a widening of the income gap between urban and rural areas and between the rich and the poor, which makes a practical difference in terms of people's ability to access medical care.

Economic development has significantly changed the dynamics of health care delivery. Prior to economic reforms, the Cooperative Medical System (CMS) provided basic health care and medicines (predominantly Western medicine) to small village clinics covering up to 90% of rural areas and constituting around 70% of the total Chinese population. The financing of CMS was derived from rural collective welfare funds, consisting of a fraction of local agricultural production or rural enterprises profits. The change in economic model resulted in the collapse of the rural collective economy[5] through financial restructuring and migration to urban areas in search of better paid jobs (which in turn caused disruption to agricultural productivity).

Since the economic reforms, most patients now have to pay privately for their medical care (for both Western and Chinese medicine) unless state, corporate or private health insurance is in place, or unless patients qualify for certain forms of social exemption, such as the exemptions for retired military personnel and civil servants. In the official statistics of 2006, over 65% of the general population had no form of health insurance, and in rural areas this was as high as 80%. Due to the cost of health care approximately, 48% of the population does not seek medical attention when it is needed, and 30% of patients opt not to stay as inpatients when it would otherwise be deemed necessary.[6] Most patients tend to delay medical attention until absolutely necessary, and in these instances the cost of treatment, such as surgery, tends to be that much greater, with a potential even to lead to family bankruptcy. Confucian medicine is still available, and at a lower cost than modern, Western-style medicine, but it is not necessarily the preferred option, although to some extent the two systems exist in parallel.

From the health care provider's point of view though, the main issue with economic reforms is an increasing focus on profitability. There are four categories of hospital in modern China: the governmental; ministerial and state-owned enterprize; military; and private share-holding hospitals. With the exception of military hospitals, which receive full governmental funding, other categories of hospital receive only partial funding, subsidy or tax exemption from central government or from the responsible ministry's health budget. The remaining funding comes from health insurance and fees paid for privately by patients, and as a result, most secondary and tertiary care centers assume responsibility for their own profits and losses.

The service provision ethos has gradually moved in recent years towards profit and sustainability. Those not covered by health insurance and who cannot afford to pay have limited or no access to health care. Physician remuneration is set at a low level, and because medical decision-making is sometimes motivated by bonus compensation from hospitals and pharmaceutical companies, this can lead to over-prescription of expensive medicines and the over-use of diagnostic and therapeutic interventions.[7]

There are clear inequalities in access and standards of care, and these are directly proportionate to consumers' purchasing power, and considerations of profitability often trump those that would be more ethical. For the richer population, the doctor-patient relationship has transformed into a literal provider-consumer relationship, whereby cost is directly proportionate to the standard of care, both perceptually by patients and in a more literal, practical sense. This means that patient autonomy may only extend as far as how much patients can afford or are willing to pay, resulting in a two-tier system, thus those who can afford it receive a better standard of care. These factors directly influence options for treatment and the choice of investigations, which poses a significant ethical challenge. Working class and low-income families are thus particular badly affected, leaving the middle and upper-middle classes to enjoy relatively comprehensive medical services.

Under this system a patient-centered approach is not universally applicable, and the implementation of Western medical ethical ideals tends to be problematic. This is not to say that the practice of medicine in China is unethical, rather that the consequences of economic reforms have made traditional ethical practices more difficult to achieve. In the end, the common moral standards of the Chinese people are still subconsciously influenced by Confucianism, and doctors who pursue benevolent actions, while both foreseeing profit and maintaining Confucian medical professionalism, are likely to be highly regarded.[8] The main issue is how state policy changes will in the future be able to redress the effects of economic reform and promote sustainable health care standards and levels of service in terms of ethical practice.

STATE POLICY ON ETHICS AND PRACTICE

The issue with virtuous practice, as traditionally advocated in China, is that practitioners inevitably differ in their personal values and in the individual degree of acceptance about what is considered virtuous. There is a state-issued code of conduct and a mechanism for accountability, but these are not entirely transparent, and the traditional ideology of "doctor knows best" is still prevalent. Very often a doctor's clinical decision plan is uncontested until the point an error occurs; therefore, as in the West, the extent to which medical decisions are ethical still depends on conscious decisions made by individual practitioners in spite of attempts by the state to be more directive.

The state has long recognized this flaw, and it adopted a paternalistic approach whereby in 1998 basic ethical standards and practice regulation were made law by the National People's Congress and the President of China. For example, the third chapter of the "Peoples Republic of China Medical Practice Act" (Clause 22.8) stipulates that all physicians must be diligent in their practice and serve to the best of their ability.[9] They must be compassionate and respectful to patients and safeguard patient confidentiality. Furthermore, they must not exploit their position to extort money from patients or suggest additional payment for their services. This code of conduct when combined with personal virtues forms a legally binding standard, and it raises physicians' accountability in terms of both ethical conduct and the law. In spite of this, however, these standards were not necessarily reflected in practice, and enforcement is not always efficient or effective.

This attempt at medical reform is largely unable to address the consequences of the economic boom in terms of increased inequalities of access to health care. However, central government has recently released new medical reform targets. There are five main areas of focus for major reforms, with an impressive timeframe for completion of three years between 2009 and 2011.[10] The most prominent and audacious plan is a basic health insurance scheme to ensure 90% coverage of the population. Other initiatives include standardizing the pricing of medicines and the elimination of reimbursement schemes provided by pharmaceutical companies for physicians and hospitals; systematic improvement of rural primary and secondary care; additional resources for a medical financial assistance system for the poor, and initiating pilot reform programs across government hospitals, with the aim of improving operations in terms of patient-centered approaches to care and improved transparency in terms of complaint procedures.

These initiatives are not only to try and counteract the issues resulting from economic reform; the ultimate goal is rapid upgrading, modernization and improvement in quality throughout the health care system. The viability and results of these targets remain to be seen, and they pose a significant test for those governing China. The reforms cover vast geographical areas, and each province has its own administrative customs, varying numbers of rich and poor, all at different stages of development in terms of economy and infrastructure.

STANDARDIZATION AND MONITORING ETHICAL PRACTICE

Amidst the government's plans to reform health care, ethical standards of practice have become legal requirements. The attainment of ethical standards in practice was inadequately addressed in previous reforms, and the government sees this aspect of the health care service as a key factor to the success of new reforms. It has recently introduced a new pilot program with an imminent plan for national implementation in the form of an ethical appraisal program that would be directly accountable to the provincial Ministry of Health.[11] All medical practitioners and allied health professionals from all types of hospitals are included, and rather like the British NHS, records of appraisal will form part of an individual's professional history.

This criteria-based appraisal system is repeated once a year, and it covers aspects of personal virtue relating to traditional Confucianism, such as compassion, patience, conscientiousness in practice, and benevolence. It also combines many key Western ethical concepts, such as informed consent and the maintenance of confidentiality. Professional attitudes and conduct are also assessed, and the appraisal consists of three parts. The self-appraisal component allows self-assessment on professional conduct, which is measured against set criteria. The second component is a workplace appraisal, consisting of other team members' impressions of an individual's performance. Thirdly, a generalized appraisal consists of a summary of patient feedback, with randomized questionnaires, including incident reports, complaints and departmental commendations.

Four grades will be awarded from the appraisal: excellent, pass, sub-standard or fail. Two consecutive sub-standard grades will constitute a fail, and practitioners receiving a failed grade, depending on the severity, would face disciplinary action that could come from either local hospital departments or the local health ministry. This process could even result in criminal prosecutions, and what will be interesting will be to see the effect these annual appraisals have on recruitment, promotion and salary banding within the respective hospitals. This system has several benefits: the three-part appraisal system would provide a reliable objective global assessment of an individual, incentives exist for individuals who perform well, and disciplinary action in cases of misconduct or sub-standard practice encourages the attainment of professional and ethical standards in clinical practice, albeit more coercively than in the West.[11]

CONCLUSION

The domination of Western medicine in China began at the turn of the 20th century, but medical ethics has remained in part Confucian. While this was culturally sustainable in the past, in recent years where economic development has sparked increasing demands for medical service, it has had a tendency to lead to tensions within the system. The economic reforms of the past 30 years have raised the living standards of the general population, but at the same time, reforms have increased the gap between rich and poor. The adoption of Western ethics has become integral to reforms and is seen as a way of maintaining standards of service.

The old welfare and medical provisions structure has been rendered ineffective with the changes in the economic model from collective farming towards a focus based on manufacturing industry and a market economy. The majority of the population has to pay for health services with little state support, and this has led to significant inequalities in terms of access and standards of care. With a health sector that is focused on profitability, ethical standards of health care delivery face new and difficult challenges. Current public health reform boldly aims at rapid change in terms of basic health care provisions, introducing a combination of enhanced legal and ethical accountability as well as a new system of State-run appraisals. These could prove to be powerful tools in helping ensure the success of reforms that have long been anticipated by the Chinese people.

REFERENCES

1. Chen MH. Confucian, Buddhist and Taoist influences on Sun SiMiao's medical ethics thoughts. *J Chinese Medical Ethics.* 2002; **15**(6): 61–2.
2. World Medical Association *Medical Ethics Manual.* 2nd ed. WMA; 2009. Available at: www.wma.net/en/30publications/30ethicsmanual/pdf/ethics_manual_en.pdf (accessed April 5, 2011).
3. MacIntrye D. *After Virtue: A study in moral theory.* 3rd rev ed. London, England: Duckworth, 2007.
4. Yang F. Influence of globalization on medical ethics in China. *J Chinese Medical Ethics.* 2001; **78**(4): 4–6.
5. Liu XZ, Yi YN. *The Health Sector in China Policy and Institutional Review.* Beijing, China: World Bank; 2004.
6. Yu X. *Blue Book of China's Society: report on quality of living in China 2005.* Beijing, China: Social Sciences Academic Press; 2006.
7. Chen XY. Defensive medicine or economically motivated corruption? A Confucian reflection on physician care in China today. *J Med Philos.* 2007; **32**(6): 635–48.
8. Fan R. Towards a Confucian virtue bioethics: reframing Chinese medical ethics in a market economy. *Theor Med Bioeth.* 2006; **27**(6): 541–66.
9. The 9th People's National Congress Assembly. *People's Republic of China Medical Practice Act 1998 [law].* Beijing, China: The People's Republic of China; 1998.
10. The Central People's Government of the People's Republic of China. *Medical, Pharmaceutical and Public Health Reform Targets 2009–2011.* Beijing, China: The People's Republic of China; 2009.
11. The State Administration of Traditional Chinese Medicine of the People's Republic of China. *Guidelines on Health care Practitioners Ethical Appraisal* [pilot]. Beijing, China: The People's Republic of China; 2007.

b) Accessing psychiatric treatment in China

Carla Marienfeld

In Chinese mythology, Shennong, also called the Yan Emperor, is the god of farming and of Chinese medicine. At a time when for most Chinese people the diet mainly consisted of animal meat, the population began to expand in a manner that could not be sustained by a meat-based diet alone. According to Chinese mythology, Shennong invented farming and taught the Chinese people how to cultivate crops. In his experiments he identified more than 70 poisonous plants in a single day, and through this process he began to create the idea that herbs and plants could cure diseases. With a medical mythology based on agriculture, rural and farming Chinese families continued to seek remedies for their illnesses in the form of herbal medication. The idea of taking a pill and then having family to provide other types of care is not new to the Chinese, and it follows in line with the way in which most modern psychiatric care is provided in China, as and when it is available.

CASE STUDY

Mr. Li is the 19-year-old son of farming minority Miao parents from a rural village in Western Hunan. He enjoys farming alongside his parents but is drawn by the dream of economic prosperity. He left home for work in a factory about one year prior to his admission to hospital. When working at the factory he became quiet and socially withdrawn from his peers, but his family attributed this to being away from the family, and in that he was performing well at the factory they were reasonably content. However, Mr. Li's sleep began to deteriorate and he felt unable to concentrate at work. He told his family he had "thoughts I don't want to think," and that these were keeping him awake at night. He felt ashamed going to work because "the others always talk about me and say bad things to me." As a result of his inability to work he was brought home back to his village. He was happy to return to his parents who took him to see a local rural doctor.

This doctor had had a total of about three years' training between Western and Chinese types of medicine since leaving school. None of his training included psychiatric disease or its treatment. Some of his traditional Chinese medicine training included ideas about emotions being linked with particular organ systems, and Mr. Li's family purchased some herbs from the doctor to treat the emotional problem that the rural doctor diagnosed. The doctor also sold them an expensive

Western medicine called *venlafaxine*, which is used to treat depression. His parents felt sure that an expensive medication must be best and that it would certainly be the most effective one available. Despite following the recommendations, Mr. Li's parents' initial concern about their son's inability to work at the factory grew into a bigger worry about his paranoia, change in demeanour and lack of concern for basic personal hygiene.

Mr. Li's family knew about the larger county hospital and sought help from there. They had no difficulty accessing care and willingly paid for the appointment (at a cost that was equivalent to less than a dollar). They were seen by a young doctor who had had five years of medical training as opposed to three; this included about 20 hours of teaching in psychiatry. He had also completed a one-year observation in internal medicine at the large university hospital prior to taking up his post at the county hospital. Noting Mr. Li's paranoia and disorganization, he listened to the family for the three minutes allotted for this appointment, during which time they explained the symptoms and asked about him hearing the voices and having strange thoughts.

The young doctor started the patient on an initial low dose of *olanzapine*, which they purchased directly from the hospital pharmacy. There was no time for questions about past medical history of the patient or his family, about other medications that he was taking or had tried, or about the social upheaval that the boy had experienced after moving away from home. No mention was made of the risks associated with the medication, whether and when it should be increased, or what to do after this one-time appointment in the outpatient clinic. Mr. Li's parents dutifully purchased the medication from the hospital pharmacy, as they had the herbs that were prescribed before, but this time it cost them roughly 60 times as much.

The parents were hopeful that their son might return to working on the farm again, and soon after that return to working in the factory. But over the next month Mr. Li grew increasingly isolated, keeping his parents awake while mumbling to himself at night. After days of badgering and asking questions, he revealed that he could "hear" his co-workers talking about him, and that one of them had implanted a computer chip in his brain to control his thoughts, monitor him and transmit their voices to him. He could not recall how or when they implanted this chip but convinced his parents that he needed medical help to remove the chip so that he could once again be at peace.

Fortunately, his parents had been able to purchase a form of health insurance, made available to rural people by the government for an annual cost of about $7. Hoping it would be to their advantage, they took a 10-hour train ride to the closest large urban city to take their son to the university hospital. They paid $1 to see the senior psychiatrist in the outpatient clinic, who had had 10 years of further education since completing medical school. They used their five minutes worth of time to explain things, and when the doctor asked the patient any questions he just stared blankly at the ground, and not making eye contact while his parents described his symptoms. The psychiatrist recommended inpatient hospitalization, a CT scan, an MRI and an EEG. Mr. Li's parents gathered the roughly $850 from extended family and personal savings to pay for the three weeks of hospitalization. This money was required prior to admission, and the parents were only likely to be able recover about 10% of the cost from their health insurance. The family signed a form indicating that they consented to involuntary hospitalization and treatment of their son, although they had little understanding about the suspected disease or the lifelong prognosis.

Mr. Li received a thorough assessment by the resident physician at the hospital, and his chart was filled in with a "history of present illness," including information about family history and past medical history, an involuntary movement scale, vital signs and basic labs, an ECG, a physical exam, and a mental status exam. Mr. Li was brought in to be interviewed by the senior physician with about 10 trainees observing. The physician asked about the auditory hallucinations, the delusions, and other symptoms of psychosis, including ideas of persecution and general paranoia, during which time Mr. Li simply sat quietly, mumbling his responses to the floor.

Soon, the 10-minute interview was completed and the patient was diagnosed with schizophrenia and put on a higher dose of *olanzapine*, as well as a medication called *sulpiride*, intended to diminish other symptoms such as lack of initiative. Mr. Li then returned to the locked unit behind a windowless large metal door, and was to attend the social skills class held by the nursing staff. He retired either to the lounge, which was filled with the noise of karaoke, or to his room, which he shared with three roommates. The physicians tried to minimize his psychotic symptoms as much as possible through a mix of medication and psychosocial rehabilitation, such as social skills training techniques, before his pre-paid time on the unit came to an end.

Mr. Li's story highlights several issues. The level of familial care illustrates a family involvement that is often cited as a reason for thinking that schizophrenia may have a better outcome in the developing world. However, this assumption is changing with new understanding that is developing regarding the complexity of this disease.[1] Eventually the patient received high quality, thorough care, but only once admitted to the inpatient unit at the university psychiatric hospital, which was on par with or even superior to similar departments that could be found in developed nations. However, as Mr. Li navigated his way from rural health care to progressively larger centers, different access and quality of care issues started to arise.

For example, questions arise about financial incentives that exist for using pharmaceutical medications, which can lead to inappropriate usage of medications. Some doctors have little education about psychiatric treatments in general, or about patient–centered approaches towards interviewing and planning treatment. This process should include patient education about the medications, with information about the risks and benefits, but difficulties in arranging follow-up sessions for patients in both outpatient and inpatient settings make this level of care difficult to achieve.

ACCESSING CARE

Many Chinese live in rural areas that tend to provide different medical services from those services that their city-dwelling peers normally enjoy.[2] Mr. Li's family initially took their concerns to a local doctor who was accessible because of his proximity and because they could afford to pay for his services directly. Concern for their son's well-being led to the family making a long and difficult journey prompted by Mr. Li's inability to work and by the family's need of his income. Patients are more likely to receive care if they show symptoms such as aggression that are harder for families to deal with in the context of rural life.[3] Because this family had the means to travel, and sufficient education about the available options for higher levels of care, they found themselves in a better situation than might otherwise have been the case.

Mr. Li's story is classic as regards the onset of schizophrenia in young males. Given the lack of education for rural doctors about mental health, and the limited extent of psychiatric education at county hospital level, it is quite possible that his symptoms could have been misunderstood or undiagnosed. In which case he could have returned to his village permanently plagued by the disability that paranoia, auditory hallucinations and delusions bring, and by anxiety from being unable to work and contribute to the well-being of the family. Most patients who gain access to the university inpatient unit have very clear, unambiguous disabling symptoms and diagnoses, but people with less clear symptoms may never be recognized as needing the interventions that could greatly improve their quality of life.

Even after obtaining care outside the rural setting, only those patients and families that recognize the need for ongoing care and have access to transportation and the time to make long journeys will have reasonable access to proper care.[5] In addition, for most people, even with health insurance plans, the financial burden of hospitalization is an expense that could only be born once, and without clearly explained plans for medication changes and/or ongoing care, there is little that can be done to deal with the side effects of any medication or uncontrollable behaviors.

PAYING FOR CARE

In the late 1970s and 1980s, the Chinese health care system changed from one that, through an elaborate network of government-supported village, county and provincial clinics, provided affordable, near-universal access to care (albeit of inconsistent quality, particularly with regard to psychiatry).[6] The newer system is a privatized, fee-for-service system, which might work reasonably well in urban settings, but with little government financial support in the rural areas, it means that it is difficult to ensure quality and consistent levels of care.[7] Private insurance companies began selling coverage in the 1980s, and following government interventions, this has recently been extended to include poorer people.[8]

Mr. Li's parents had a form of insurance that would reimburse 10% of their costs, but members of family and others from his rural farming village were required to pre-pay his hospital stay prior to the patient receiving care. In a short time the expectation of access to health care that arises from being a Chinese citizen has given way to general acceptance of a system whereby everything has to be paid for when it is needed with little or no government support. When citizens discuss the role of their government in ensuring the economic success of the country, there seems to be a hopeful attitude about progress wherein health care, human rights, and other rights associated with a higher standard of living will follow with economic success. China has seen a growth of its middle classes, who are able to afford to see doctors, purchase private health insurance, and pay for their medications.[9] However, this situation is mostly limited to those living in large urban areas.

Thirty years before, the government would have paid the doctors' salary in the smaller clinics and provided support for the hospitals.[10] Health care providers now gain income directly from carrying out procedures and tests, and from selling prescription medicines. As hospital income increases by virtue of these arrangements, hospital staff now receive bonuses. This creates potential disincentives for using limited, cost-effective recommendations.[11] In smaller facilities where the low cost of seeing a doctor does not inhibit access, income to support the clinic comes mainly from medications that are sold, and limitations exist in terms of what families can afford and the consistent availability of medications.

Mr. Li was started on *olanzapine*, which is a newer antipsychotic medication. In the past, a patient with schizophrenia was more likely to have been on *clozapine*, which is one of few anti-psychotics that has evidence for its superiority, is cheap and is not restricted in China by concerns about the rare blood disorders that have been associated with its use.[12] While *clozapine* is still widely used in China, and because of the incentives, Mr. Li is now more likely than in the past to be given an expensive antipsychotic drug, which is no more efficacious than older ones and has equally worrisome side effects.

As in some settings in the West, educational material about antipsychotic drugs is provided to teaching physicians, complete with the drug company's logo. There are drug advertisements on hallway placards, pens/boxes in interview spaces bearing brand names of pharmaceutical products, and free samples that are generally widely available. The drug companies fund facilities as well as trips to international academic meetings for physicians. In addition, a free-market system of drug provision in China is leading to reduced availability of the older and effective medications that have become so cheap that distributors can no longer afford to provide them.[13] Observations showed that trainees receive little education about the bias in design of many pharmaceutical-supported studies, or about information bias in the literature that they distribute. As in the West, students in China are not always taught how to critically evaluate the sources of the information that they are given.

COST VERSUS QUALITY

With the introduction of Western products, pop culture and business practices that arrived with China's economic boom came an increased acceptance and even expectation of Western medicines, as opposed to the simple reliance on traditional Chinese medicines. There seems to be acceptance amongst patients that a combination of the two types of medicine works well, even though the balance is now shifting between them because of the prominent place enjoyed by Western-style pharmaceutical companies. Amongst physicians at the university hospital, the belief seems to be that Chinese medicines and herbs provide comfort, ritual and a sense of continuity to patients who demand them, whereas Western medicines are the ones that "actually help patients." The fact that Western medicines are provided by the highly trained physicians at the larger urban centers adds to the perception that they are seen as being high quality, and modern medicines are gradually taking the place of traditional, folk medicines.

In the minds of patients, the high cost that people have to pay in order to obtain these medicines correlates with a sense of their increased worth. The transition from government-provided care to a system incorporating private health insurance seems to add to this perception, supporting the idea that the more you pay then the better quality care that you receive. Consistent with the founding myths of medicine that exist in China, much of what is expected from a non-surgical doctor's visit involves nothing more than the provision of medications. In paying for the *olanzapine*, Mr Li's parents faithfully accepted the premise that, partly because of high cost, this is the best quality treatment.

With little education about the illness, alternative treatment options or significant risks associated with this pharmaceutical medication, the decisions Mr. Li's family took were based almost solely on the physician's recommendation. While the newest and best medications are seen as priority in seeking care from a physician, patients also want to spend time with their doctor. In order to achieve this they are even prepared to fight to secure a place in the first-come, first-served queue at the outpatient psychiatric clinic at a university hospital. Families expect that their $1 will buy them a brief window of time so that skilled ears can listen to their concerns and provide the expertise to find them the exact medication they need in order to try and reduce their suffering.

The families rush to cram in every detail they can whilst the psychiatrist listens or interrupts them to ask key questions and write the prescription, or to advise them on hospitalization. Visits can be interrupted by other patients wanting to ensure their place in the line, with little regard to privacy or to the subject matter being discussed. Despite the time allowed for the exchange of information and the time available for education about the diagnosis, prognosis and the medication side effects, there is still much faith in the physician. Families dutifully pay for the expensive prescriptions and see that the patient takes his medication, whether or not patients are aware of what it is they are taking. Issues around patient consent are barely even considered.

CONCERNS ABOUT MEDICATION AND CORRECT DOSE

Mr. Li was initially started on *venlafaxine*, a medication that is most often used for depression. When seen in rural clinics, decisions about medication are made based on what is available in the town and what the family can afford. Availability, in turn, is influenced by the site of manufacturing, distribution and marketing by the drug company. For example, herbal remedies prepared locally are often available inexpensively, although now, even traditional Chinese medicine remedies are produced and marketed on a large scale. In the case of Western drugs, a patient may have access to medications in a local clinic, but it is unlikely that all classes and types will be available to be given when a correct diagnosis has been made.[14] Perhaps Mr. Li was given *venlafaxine* because it was known to be available in the clinic and known to be used for some type of emotional problems. In addition, most psychiatric medications should be started off at low dosages and then increased based on the patient's tolerability. Given a lack of systematic follow-up care, it is common for patients to remain on starter doses and for them never to be increased. This was the case with the *olanzapine* Mr. Li was given; the usual starting dose is 5 mg per day, whereas the normal dosage to treat paranoia and psychotic symptoms is between 10–15 mg.

QUESTIONS OF EDUCATION AND EXPERIENCE

Mr. Li was fortunate to have been seen by doctors who recognized his symptoms as being emotional and/or psychiatric in origin, and he was referred for higher levels of care by physicians who had successively greater levels of training. Many doctors in rural settings are unlikely to have had more than a few years of medical training, and often they have no training about mental health, despite the prevalence and enormous burden that these diseases inflict worldwide.[15] With improved and standardized training about mental health diagnosis and treatment, Mr. Li could have been diagnosed much earlier and started on an appropriate medication to treat the symptoms of schizophrenia. The care he received in the university hospital inpatient unit was provided by a combination of highly educated physicians with upwards of 10 years or more postgraduate education and experience, as well as trainees that were eager to apply their knowledge and education. The emphasis on psychosocial rehabilitation techniques in the inpatient setting was also state of the art.

SUMMARY

Mr. Li, a factory worker from a rural farming community in central China, was able to find his way to psychiatric care. While he initially had easy access to care, limited knowledge and treatment options placed restrictions on the utility of this care. His family's faith in doctors and the curative potential of medications, as well as the impairment caused to them by his disease/behavior, led them from the countryside through increasing layers of care in terms of quality to his ultimate hospitalization. Although schizophrenia is often a chronic illness, given the expense and the distance, this will almost certainly be his last hospitalization, regardless of whether he needs further treatment. Mr. Li will return to his family with better-controlled symptoms and some pills, and the tradition of Chinese medicine continues, based on use of a prescription, with the family providing ancillary care for anything that medication cannot cure.

[*The paper is based on personal interviews and the direct experiences of the contributor, drawn from a period of time spent observing a psychiatric facility at a large urban university hospital in Changsha, Hunan Province, China.*]

REFERENCES

1. Cohen A, Patel V, Thara R, Gureje O. Questioning an axiom: better prognosis for schizophrenia in the developing world? *Schizophr Bull.* 2008; **34**(2): 229–44.
2. Liu TQ, Ng C, Ma H, *et al.* Comparing models of mental health service systems between Australia and China: implications for the future development of Chinese mental health service. *Chin Med J (Engl).* 2008; **121**(14); 1331–8.
3. Ibid.
4. Wang, X. [*Informal interview.*] Changsha, China. November 9, 2008.
5. Tan C, Shinfuku N, Sim K. Psychotropic prescription practices in east Asia: looking back and peering ahead. *Curr Opin Psychiatry.* 2008; **21**(6): 645–50.
6. Ibid.
7. Liu, op. cit.
8. Wang, op. cit.
9. Xiao, S. [Informal interview.] Changsha, China. November 2008.
10. Ibid.
11. Liu, op. cit.
12. Tan, op. cit.
13. Liu, Z. [Informal interview.] Changsha, China. November 2008.
14. Xiao, op. cit.
15. Prince M, Patel V, Saxena S, *et al.* No health without mental health. *The Lancet.* 2007; **370**(9590): 859–77.

CHAPTER 6

Medicine, ethics and professionalism in modern India

a) Indian philosophy and bioethics

Roger Worthington

Ethics is concerned with the moral basis of how people conduct their lives, and Indian philosophy has much to offer in this regard, as it has a very ancient tradition. While the modern bioethics movement may have begun in America in the second half of the 20th century, ethical thought did not begin there any more than it did in Greece with Hippocrates or with Aristotle around 400 BCE. Ethical thought is closely associated with aphoristic teachings from the Himalayas, and while this is not the time nor place to explore these sources, modern bioethics can learn from examining classical Indian philosophical roots. The philosophy of yoga, for instance, is rich in references to the nature and quality of people's thoughts and actions, and such insights could potentially provide an underpinning that is sometimes seen as lacking in the modern bioethics movement.

While bioethics and religion have links, they do not extend to include institutional religion, and if the word "ethics" is prefixed by descriptors such as Jewish, Catholic, Hindu, Buddhist or Islamic, it can clearly influence the nature and content of what is discussed. While morality and human values have a universality that goes beyond social, cultural and geographical divisions, the way in which issues are addressed differs according to time and place as well as the way in which the issues themselves are analyzed. Limiting ethics to discourse within a single religious framework cannot be seen as "morally wrong," but it is different from studying ethics "qua ethics," whether theoretical or applied.

India as a country has all of the above—a Hindu majority, large Muslim and Jain minorities, plus adherents to many other religions as well as those who profess no religious affinity. The last category is slightly different in India from what it might be in the West because religion tends to define cultural heritage to a greater extent in India, irrespective of whether it is formally practiced.

Putting religion aside, ethics, law and medicine have complex interrelations, and careful analysis is needed to see how they work and how they are relevant to modern medical practice. This applies to India no less than to anywhere else, and while the country may have strong spiritual and philosophical traditions, not everyone in India is brought up in accordance with these traditions or is actively incorporating them into their daily lives.

In that relationships between ethics, law and medicine are dynamic and fluid, when rapid change occurs in society, such as is happening in 21st century India, this has the potential to lead to a reappraisal of what in moral terms society is willing to accept. If one understands morals in a normative sense as referring to social customs that society considers acceptable, then it is both logical and self-evident that moral standards will evolve over time. While there is no reason to doubt that ethics plays a role within professional practice in India, the one it currently plays is neither well defined nor highly regarded, either in practice settings or in relation to medical education.[1,2]

MODERN CODES

For some physicians there is an expectation that a person committed to a profession such as medicine simply ought to be behave in a certain way, which may explain why the formal teaching of ethics and law plays only a relatively minor part in the practice of medicine in modern India. While codes issued by the Medical Council of India[3] are consistent with standards set by bodies such as the World Medical Association,[4] ethical codes are only as good as the systems that support their implementation. Without effective regulatory systems, ethical codes are little more than exercises in public relations, thus having little or no practical relevance to patient care.

There is an apparent dichotomy between balancing on the one hand the need for consistent standards to be applied across the profession, and on the other, respecting the rights and religious freedoms of individuals, which perhaps are nowhere cherished more strongly than they are in India. There may be no neat, simple solution to deciding how this balance should be achieved, and it is logically incoherent and ethically problematic for a physician to work solely according to his or her own personal code of practice. By definition, standard-setting has to have broad terms of reference; however, in India the more individualistic approach to standards is probably the one that prevails overall. Therefore, what this means for patient care depends on who is doing the treating as much as on what formal codes might be in place.

Applying codes in relation to personal beliefs and convictions is one thing, but forcing beliefs on to others is something else, and contrary to international norms in terms of agreed codes of professional practice. An interesting case that highlights this question concerns a British Muslim dentist who refused to treat female Muslim patients unless they were wearing the "hijab" (Islamic headdress) when attending for treatment at his clinic. Following complaints from patients, the case ultimately led to the regulatory authority reaching a judgment of serious professional misconduct.[5] Duty of care can and does trump individual beliefs, especially if expressed coercively. There may be times when health care professionals should discharge responsibility for treating a patient by referring that person on to another qualified professional. If conscience makes it impossible to treat a particular patient (which in this case meant a woman with a bare head), there must be a degree of reasonableness and responsibility, both of which were lacking in this case.

When it comes to issues of probity and working with patients and colleagues, guidance in the UK states that "you must make sure that your conduct at all times justifies your patients' trust in you and the public's trust in the profession."[6] Fulfilling such a requirement requires more than simply adhering to a set of rules, and how this might apply in India is something worth considering. Adherence to formal codes means two things: firstly that codes must have been agreed, and secondly, that mechanisms must be in place for upholding those standards. One without the other has little relevance, and therefore when discussing probity and professionalism in India important questions arise:

1 Is there any reason why standards of professional probity should not apply in India?
2 What happens if anything to a doctor if these standards are not adhered to?
3 Finally, to what extent does it matter given other challenges that exist towards the provision of health care in a country the size of India?

The first answer must surely be "no." India has signed up to international protocols and is a member of the World Health Organization, and whatever challenges the country faces, there is no valid reason why ethical standards upholding professionalism and probity should not apply. The practice of medicine is based on trust wherever it is practiced, and without this trust the doctor-patient relationship cannot function effectively. Public trust in the profession is as important as trust in an individual clinician treating a particular patient; therefore, when one reads about "the rot within" the Medical Council of India, which is the national regulatory body, there is reason to be concerned.[7]

The paper to which reference is being made describes serious failings at a high level that are serious enough to cause one to ask whether standards of professionalism and probity are being upheld at all. If this is the case then everything is going to be down to individual clinicians to maintain appropriate standards when performing their duties, with or without effective regulatory frameworks. The medical profession is hierarchical in the way that it works in most countries around the world, including India, and it is well known that junior doctors tend to follow patterns of behavior set by their seniors. Therefore, if these standards are not upheld, the effect can filter down and cause systemic failings. That this has already started happening is a matter of serious concern, and there are signs of corruption having made inroads into the profession.[8]

While answers to the second question (about what happens to a doctor who does not meet set standards) will depend on circumstances, if the answer is "nothing," one has to question the point of setting standards at all. In order for standards to be taken seriously they must be taught and followed, even allowing for pragmatic considerations. Evidence suggests that this is not currently happening in modern India, and ethics and professionalism are not taught routinely to either medical students or trainees.[9,10] Given concerns about the lead regulatory body, clinicians may *have* to work to their own personal standards of professionalism, which has the potential to result in inconsistencies and a low common denominator in terms of standards. The strong possibility exists that ethical standards, as defined by international agreement, are simply ignored, which is not a good conclusion to have to reach.

As regards the third question (does it matter?), consequences exist whether seen or unseen, immediate or long-term, that affect the clinician as well as the patient. It matters whether or not a doctor behaves in a certain way; clinical and ethical standards go hand in hand, and sub-standard clinical care inherently fails to show proper respect for patients, which can in turn impact on patient outcomes. Unethical conduct, for example, whether forging signatures, giving or taking bribes, plagiarizing on an exam or ignoring patients' rights, has the potential to put patients at risk. If nobody intervenes, bad practices will continue to go unchecked.

Ethical and professional standards are certain to vary to some extent in India because the country is large and because many organizations work at state as opposed to national level. This applies equally to health and the law, and there may well not be consistency, for example, between Kerala in the south and Uttarakhand in the north in terms of jurisprudence. From an ethical standpoint this need not matter as long as the different systems work effectively and are broadly compatible in relation to national standards. This much ought to be a realistic and achievable goal, even though there is reason to think that this is not the case.[11]

PATIENT AND PHYSICIAN PERSPECTIVES

To take another perspective, patient expectations may differ, and it could simply be that a patient's primary concern is merely to be seen by a physician. If in order to achieve this, patients and their families have to travel great distances, then ethical standards of conduct might even be viewed as an unaffordable luxury.

But this would be a worrying conclusion because very sick patients are always vulnerable, and there might be few viable options that are available. If the lives of patients rest in the hands of a doctor who has little regard for ethical standards, then it is especially important to have mechanisms in place that can help to protect patients.

This means there should be effective ways of promoting safeguards and penalizing doctors who significantly fail to demonstrate and uphold proper standards of care. Ethics and professionalism should never be an "unaffordable luxury," and the public needs to be assured that members of the medical profession will behave in an appropriate and safe way. If ethics and morals are effectively the same, and if ethics and professionalism go together, which it would seem they do, then professionalism and morality *must* go hand in hand.

This is potentially difficult when clinicians have beliefs and principles that differ significantly between one individual and another, and so the paradox has not gone away. In a pluralist multi-cultural society such as India's, where religion is still a determining influence in many people's lives, an inclusive approach to standard-setting is crucial. Ethical values need to be set in broad terms, even though social and legal context will make a difference when it comes to the more practical considerations. In the final analysis, there is a balance to be achieved in terms of where personal standards of belief begin and end, and where national and international standards will apply and trump those beliefs. *How* physicians perceive ethics is as important as the place ethics and professionalism hold in society as a whole. If in India these are seen as being simply matters of personal and private morality, then this can be problematic. There is good reason to think that professional standards ought to be openly discussed, agreed, taught and then implemented, and in that order. This conclusion would seem to be inescapable.

b) Health care in the Himalayas

It is time to move now from the abstract to the applied in terms of underlying ethics. At the practical level, difficulties can arise when it comes to health care service provision in physically remote communities (in India no less than in other countries). The geography of a region such as the mid-Himalayas gives rise to real and practical constraints. For example, a patient needing to see a doctor may have to make a journey taking several hours, and if only one bus a day goes between towns and villages, e.g. between Mukteshwar, which is a village 7,500 feet up above sea level, and Nainital, which is a medium-sized town high in the foothills in the province of Uttarakhand, it could take two days complete the journey—with an overnight stay in between—in order for a patient to be able to attend clinic and receive necessary care.

This has economic implications for families and patients; such constraints serve as deterrents to receiving treatment, which in turn leads to medical conditions not being treated when they should be, or to their not being treated at all. This gives rise to increased risks of both morbidity and mortality. Patients needing hospitalization or major surgical intervention can have even further to travel to reach a big city; also, in monsoon times, roads are often blocked by landslides, and during times of religious festival, roads are sometimes impassable due to hoards of pilgrims traveling on foot, even on major highways. These difficulties mean that the sickest patient can find it especially hard to make a long journey, and the poor physical condition of the roads brings added difficulties in terms of travel. Monsoons will continue, as will religious festivals, and so while roads could be improved, these factors in combination add up to a set of circumstances that can affect decisions about whether, where and when a patient receives medical treatment.

In India good quality medical care can best be accessed in major cities, provided one can pay and/or one has adequate private health insurance. But for those who have neither and who live outside the cities, this could mean traveling and spending days camping in the grounds of a state hospital, waiting to be seen by a physician. For people living in villages in remote mountain communities, viable options for receiving anything other than basic care remain limited. Public-private partnerships are beginning to be seen in India, in which support is provided by central government in return for providing services to those unable to afford treatment or medical insurance.

While state-run hospitals exist in all major cities, the mismatch between supply and demand is probably unbridgeable because of the size of the country, the low level of earnings in rural areas, and the small number of publicly funded hospitals. The partnership model may be the only one that will be able to lessen this gap, and while it is too soon to know what impact these public-private partnerships will have in terms of improved access, the initial evidence is regrettably not promising.[12]

There is an added difficulty when viewed from the doctor's perspective, because there are few incentives for doctors to go and work in the remote rural areas. Doctors in such places tend to have low rates of pay, and for reasons due to geography they are unable to commute to tap into better-paid work in the cities. This often leaves rural communities having to manage with little by way of health care amenities and provision. Doctors who do agree to work in remote areas cannot afford to provide properly for their families, being in receipt of only small, state-supported salaries; in addition, they have only limited access to modern medical technology.

In India as in other countries, the divide between rich and poor and urban and rural is large and growing, giving rise to increased difficulty in terms of fair access and the distribution of scarce resources. However, there have been some recent developments, and in terms of improved health care access, the government of Uttarakhand recently started an emergency service, similar to "999" in the UK or "911" in the USA, although this fledgling service comes with its own problems.

The closest emergency station to Mukteshwar is a least an hour away, and it is only able to deal with a small number of calls. For example, on one occasion, an English doctor working in the region on behalf of a local charity was told when a particular emergency arose that no medically trained person was able to come and attend. Only after speaking directly to the medical officer in charge was it agreed that someone would attend within two hours.

There are further limitations to this service, such as limited staff training and certain types of equipment and drugs that are simply not available. For example, on another occasion, the oxygen supply did not work, and on another there were insufficient supplies of the drug atropine that was to be used to treat a case of pesticide poisoning. The service only provides transport to take people to a hospital; it is up to patients and families to fund the hospital stay and to pay for the necessary drugs (as well as the journey home).

There are a few alternatives in terms of where and how people are able to access health care. One source of care is at the local level from village healers, who conduct religious ceremonies for particular diseases (such as jaundice, possibly secondary to hepatitis A, which is rife in the region during monsoon time). But this type of care would depend on the religious practice of the healer as well as on the religion of the person wanting to be healed. Another potential source of help is available from local pharmacists, who do have some basic training and who are usually well established in the community and therefore trusted, especially in treating minor ailments. However, they tend to prescribe drugs without either seeing patients or examining them. Furthermore, pharmacists' remuneration is dependent upon how many medicines are sold, which can lead to common drugs such as steroids and antibiotics being overprescribed.

Various Non-Governmental Organizations (NGOs) work within the region, but doctors often come and go and it is difficult for NGOs to find reliable staff who are willing to stay for the longer term. Patients lose confidence in services if they are uncertain about who or what will be there next time that they need medical help. There is also variability in terms of training for staff supplied by the NGOs, with no established protocols and no system for implementing agreed-upon standards of care. Since patients have to pay for consultations and treatment sometimes they choose only to see the pharmacist if it means having access to free consultations. In cases where there is a serious medical problem, it could in the end save money to travel to see a doctor in the city, as the person there would be better trained. At the local level, some people perceive that the NGOs are corrupt, leading to a further erosion of confidence in services as and when they are available.

Government village workers provide services, but these are mostly concerned with preventative medicine. These workers, who have a basic level of training in diagnosing and providing treatments, are linked with local hospitals, making it possible for them to organize referrals. These village workers have a stock of basic medicines, which they are able to provide free of charge, and this is a major consideration when local wages generally are low. Government hospitals, however, are associated with long wait times, as well as with variable standards of care and high-cost medicines. Besides questions of accessibility, these hospitals tend to be poorly viewed by people in local communities.

There are private hospitals and private doctors in the cities that offer high-quality, high-cost services to those who can afford them. Families vary in terms of who they decide to consult, depending on the perceived cause of illness and its severity, as well as on their financial resources. This choice is also linked to levels of education, and it would be a family decision about who to consult; it is not just a matter of individual choice. For example, older men tend to have better access to health care than younger women, even if they come from the same family, because of traditional customs and practices and variation in education levels of achievement, i.e. access is influenced by gender and age.

Families may decide to switch from one source of help to another if options offered by one are either not believed or are not practical. To take an actual example, a mother brought her 5-year-old daughter to see a doctor in Bhowali, which involved undertaking a significant journey. The daughter had persistent bleeding and bruising, and the doctor did some basic investigations before telling them that this was a serious condition and that they would have to go to Delhi for further investigation and treatment. This was another very long journey, and the family said that it was not something they could afford. After waiting approximately 10 months without treatment, the girl started bleeding severely from her nose. The village healer was called to assist because the family was unhappy with the treatment being offered by the local medical doctor, and they sought no other formal help. The condition of the girl started to deteriorate. She died just two days after the bleeding started at home, and the cause of the bleeding was never investigated.

At a policy level, there is a new government initiative to encourage or even coerce newly qualified doctors to go and work in remote areas for a year. This will not be popular with the doctors, and it may not provide continuity of care in terms of patients being able to see the same person over time; however, if it works, the plan ought to make a difference and significantly improve access to medical care in the rural areas. What follows next is a practical example of some of the complexities and obstacles that lie in the way of effective service provision.

CASE EXAMPLE

A woman was in labor at home and a nurse and charity-funded doctor had been called to attend the birth. She had hypertension in late pregnancy, but because she had no symptoms she and her family did not appreciate why this needed to be investigated and therefore it was not. At her house the early stages of labor progressed normally, but because of high blood pressure and the increased risk this brings to the mother and child, a decision was made to transfer her to the local hospital, only after due deliberation with her husband and father-in-law. The woman in this case has few autonomous rights and it would be unacceptable for her to give consent without first consulting with male members of the family to ask permission and to consider the question of who will pay for any treatment.

After an hour's walk, the party of four (the woman in labor, her husband, the nurse and the attending doctor) arrived at the hospital, by which time the labor had progressed further. After another hour she was fully dilated and her membranes had ruptured but then there was no further progress and it became clear that the labor was obstructed. A decision was made by the medical and nursing team to transfer the patient as a matter of urgency to the nearest obstetric center. The husband was told this, but he wished to wait and see what would happen, as his family had no money to pay for the transfer.

After a further period of waiting and no progress with the delivery, the husband walked home to ask permission from his father, who also needed to be consulted and who was not available by telephone. This necessitated going down mountain roads in the dark and then back up again; only when he returned and gave permission was it possible to call the ambulance. After a further period of waiting the ambulance arrived, and everyone drove down to Bhowali (the closest town with proper hospital facilities). By this time the baby's head was almost out, and the hospital staff managed to deliver the baby, who then needed to be transferred to a neonatal unit in another town. The family is glad because the baby is a boy and alive and well, but they had to pay for the five-day stay at the neonatal unit. Eventually the group, including the medical and nursing team, returned to Mukteshwar at five o'clock in the morning, this time on a milk float, not in an ambulance. Such are some of the medical care realities in this remote mountain region of northern India (*see* endnote p. 152).

REFERENCES

1. Chattopadhyay S. Teaching Ethics in an Unethical Setting: "Doing nothing" is neither good nor right. *Indian J Med Ethics.* 2009; 6(2): 93–6. Available at: www.issuesinmedicalethics.org/172co93.html (accessed August 4, 2009).
2. Mahajan V. White-coated corruption. *Indian J Med Ethics.* 2010; 7(1): 18–20.
3. Medical Council of India. Codes of Ethics Regulations 2002 (amended 2010). Available at: www.mciindia.org/RulesandRegulations/CodeofMedicalEthicsRegulations2002.aspx (accessed March 25, 2011).
4. World Medical Association International Code of Medical Ethics. Available at: www.wma.net/en/30publications/10policies/c8/index.html (accessed March 25, 2011).
5. The Telegraph. *Muslim NHS dentist 'tried to force patients to wear traditional Islamic dress.'* London: July 2, 2009. Available at: www.telegraph.co.uk/news/newstopics/religion/5718982/Muslim-NHS-dentist-tried-to-force-patients-to-wear-traditional-Islamic-dress.html (accessed August 5, 2009).
6. General Medical Council (UK). *Good Medical Practice.* 2006 [§ 57]. Available at: www.gmc-uk.org/guidance/good_medical_practice/index.asp (accessed July 27, 2009).
7. Pandya SK. Medical council of India: the rot within. *Indian J Med Ethics.* 2009; 6(3): 125–31.
8. Mahajan, op. cit.
9. Thomas G. *Medical Council of India and the Indian Medial Association: uneasy relations. Indian J Med Ethics.* 201; 8(1): 2. Available at: www.issuesinmedicalethics.org/191ed2.html (accessed March 25, 2011).
10. Ravindran GD. Medical ethics education in India. *Indian J Med Ethics.* 2008; 5(1): 18–19. Available at: www.issuesinmedicalethics.org/magic/articletemplate.rhtml?iss=161co18.html&prn=yes (accessed August 4, 2009).
11. Pandya, op. cit.
12. Thomas G, Krishnan S. Effective public-private partnership in healthcare: Apollo as a cautionary tale. *Indian J Med Ethics.* 2010; 7(1): 2–4.

CHAPTER 7

Health and social policy trends in Malaysia

Noor Sulastry Yurni Ahmad

BACKGROUND

Malaysia has an emerging multi-sector economy and a two-tier system for delivering health care services: a government-led and funded public sector, and a thriving private sector. Malaysia has good health indicators and a generally accessible health system, which is primary care led. However, as yet, Malaysia does not have a unified system of health care that provides every citizen with universal access. The public sector caters for the bulk of the population (about 65%), but it is only served by about 45% of registered doctors and even fewer specialists (25–30%). Furthermore, a heavily subsidized public sector is almost entirely funded by central government, with patients paying only nominal fees for outpatient care and hospitalization. The private sector, on the other hand, has grown significantly over the past 25 years, giving rise to questions about the sustainability of the present arrangements.

In the half-century since independence in 1957, the health care system in Malaysia developed well, and government-provided services currently enjoy a good measure of popular support. Even Malaysian people living in village areas are able to seek medical and health services from government centers via public rural clinics (known as *klinik desa*). People in urban areas have ready access to public health services, and periodic upgrading of the rural health service program has contributed to its continuing relevance. Furthermore, the government continues to support hospitals that provide a range of primary, secondary and tertiary care in urban areas, meaning that these facilities provide higher levels of care than those in rural clinics.

Although the private sector played a significant role in the evolution of the health care system, the government of Malaysia still plays the major role as it monitors health care provision, benchmarking it against local services in the private sector. In recent years the private health sector has become increasingly well-developed, making it necessary to consider the introduction of a form of national health insurance. For example, major university hospitals previously run by the government have now been privatized, and the remaining teaching hospitals are expected to follow suit. The medical store (in Petaling Jaya) that previously produced and distributed medicines to government health facilities has also been privatized, and the National Heart Institute (Institut Jantung Negara) similarly functions as a corporate entity.[1]

In addition to providing medical care, private firms provide support services to government hospitals, and with growing levels of corporatization, the government hopes the burden of financing health care services will gradually decrease. In the last 10 years the government has been reluctant to put adequate resources into health care services and to improve remuneration and working conditions to a high enough level as to be able to retain a full range of specialist health professionals. Nonetheless, full integration of private-public health care sectors appears unlikely, and better partnership collaborations are now the goal, in which the best of each system is meant to be retained.

A United Nations Human Development Report (2006) ranks Malaysia as 61st in the world; in the same year the World Health Report stated that the Malaysian government spends 6.9% of gross domestic product on health care. However, even these relatively modest levels of health care spending are in doubt as the government considers the sustainability of its spending over the longer term.

MALAYSIAN SOCIAL POLICY

The Malaysian government reviewed health care financing in 1983, and one of the key recommendations was to set up a national health security fund as an alternative source of financing for health care services. More recently, according to the Seventh Malaysia Plan, the government intends to set up a National Health Security Fund (NHSF), and Malaysia is one of few developing countries to have guided its post-independence development strategy using national development plans. The Seventh Malaysia Plan (1996–2000), which was the ninth in a series of five-year plans, was released just before the onset of the 1997–99 economic crisis that put an end to a nine-year economic boom. The crisis dramatically changed the economic landscape of the country, requiring an overhauling of the plan for economic recovery following on from a deep recession.

There has always been an overarching concern for the common citizen, especially with regard to poorer segments of Malaysian society, and this has broadly led to the development of a social contract model based on health care entitlements and rights. There exists a deep-seated commitment on the part of the Malaysian government to try and eradicate poverty and to encourage development of human social capital. As a result, the government tries to take up the shortfall for unexpected costs arising from catastrophic illness or injury as well as for the provision of services for treating chronic disease.[3]

DEVELOPMENTS AND STRUCTURES
OF THE MALAYSIAN HEALTH CARE SYSTEM

The national Malaysian health care system is publicly funded, and it was set up to emphasize efficiency, rationality and socially just principles of health care. This is regulated according to accountable and transparent criteria, and the system tries to be flexible. The government could continue to provide existing services in addition to maintaining a regulatory role in a mixed public-private health care system,[4] but the steady decline of public funded health care is becoming a reality. This is in spite of the fact that the public sector performed well in delivering primary health care to the majority of the population at reasonable cost.

The government introduced a new patient fee-paying system in 2005 known as the full-paying patient (FPP) scheme, whereby part of the fees paid are used directly for physicians' reimbursement to supplement their earnings. For those willing and able to pay, this scheme offers ready access to services and shorter waiting times for elective surgeries and other therapies than would otherwise be voluntary. There were fears that this scheme would encourage queue-jumping and penalize the poor, and consumer pressure groups called for its abandonment.[5] However, both sectors play a role in determining access and equality of health care provision, and the largest sector in terms of public service provision is in rural health care services.[6] The government provides almost all the infrastructure and human resources such as doctors, nurses, pharmacists, dentists and allied health professionals at various local centers.

Resources are distributed to various parts of the country based on the size and needs of populations in different districts and states. However, problems occur in remote areas; places that are hardly accessible because they are either river-bound or simply jungle (such as Perak, Pahang, Sabah and Sarawak). Government deployment of health professionals to these rural areas is unpopular, and remote locations discourage health professionals from helping to deliver medical services in these areas because it is financially unrewarding. Professionals expect to enjoy a certain standard of living, and they want government to offer them more incentives to help professionals provide the same level of services to patients as would be the case for people living in less remote areas. At present there are no incentives for the private sector to become involved in delivering health care services in these remote rural locations.[7]

In terms of urban health, a rise in private health care was seen in the 1980s, and private hospital beds increased from around 5–25% in terms of the private sector's share.[8] This sector employs around 55% of all registered doctors, but these same doctors only look after about 25% of the population. This represents an inequitable distribution of a limited resource in the form of skilled, experienced health professionals. Most doctors only choose to work in one sector or the other, and without recourse to coercion or greater government incentives, there is no simple solution to this problem.

Within the private sector most patients are self-paying, using fee-for-service arrangements; however, third-party involvement is increasingly becoming the norm via private health insurance arrangements.[9] Interestingly, both political and practical factors have restrained the government from introducing wider privatization policies within the health sector.[10] Any radical change in the role of the state as a health care provider poses problems of political legitimacy for a ruling coalition that projects itself as delivering socioeconomic benefits to the whole population, including to its principal constituents, who are the rural Malays.

Despite a strong commitment to the privatization of state enterprises and services, the government has so far only introduced a selective degree of privatization into the health sector, in spite of pronouncements to the contrary. Hemodialysis, pharmaceutical distribution and hospital support services have all largely been transferred to the private sector, but moves to privatize public hospital services further is generating opposition from a range of interest groups, some of whom are demanding a role in public policymaking. Government may need to make greater efforts to engage in public debate and to explain to the public the future direction of the health policy. In nearby Singapore a model of corporate health care practice shows a tried and tested scheme that works and that is capable of responding to the diverse health care needs of a population.[11] However, Singapore offers a very different model from the two-strand model that currently exists in Malaysia, and in order for a fully private health care system to work in Malaysia there would need to be a sea change in terms of public opinion.

WOMEN'S HEALTH

Malaysia aims to become a fully developed nation by the year 2020, and women's health care priorities are set to change. Programs put in place to provide reproductive medical care and to ensure the survival of women and young children need to be able to cope with other emerging issues in terms of women's health. Many Malaysian women are now overweight or suffer from obesity and from the effects of lifestyles that were usually associated with men, such as smoking and unhealthy sexual behavior. Women's health programs that focus on wellness and lifestyle approaches to health are now trying to provide a broader range of services for women.[12]

In terms of social patterns, Malaysian women are in some respects in an advantageous position, and efforts made by government are yielding positive results. For example, more girls are now enrolled in tertiary education, women are more often empowered to make their own decisions, females are fast gaining in economic independence and they increasingly participate in all spheres of life. But these essential beginnings need to expand in order to safeguard and improve the health of Malaysian women in the future. Modern attitudes and changes in relation to women's role in society, coupled with changing perceptions regarding the maintenance of low body weight, have resulted in higher rates of women smoking. This increasing prevalence has been conceded by the Ministry of Health, and habits will need to change in the future if government efforts aimed at trying to reduce the numbers of women smokers are going to work. Pamphlets have started to appear from the Ministry of Health on the effects of passive smoking, portraying the wives of male smokers as being victims.

The government recognizes the problem with women smokers, citing the bad example given to children by parents who choose to smoke. The government permitted tobacco companies to take part in campaigns to discourage youth from smoking, and gender sensitivity is evident in a new program designed by the Confederation of Malaysian Tobacco Manufacturers that discourages underage smoking.[13] In addition, a cross-sectional study was conducted on female students enrolled in private higher learning institutions in Kuala Lumpur and Selangor in Malaysia in 2005. It identified risk factors that could be used to develop more effective prevention programs to overcome smoking among young urban women.[14]

The Asian-Pacific Resource and Research Centre for Women (ARROW) was established in 1993 as a regional, non-governmental, non-profit women's organization based in Kuala Lumpur. The centre, funded by international aid agencies, focuses on women's health in general and reproductive health in particular. ARROW provides a number of women-only and family health programs. These include family planning, cancer screening, adolescent health care, HIV screening (including antenatal screening), anti-retroviral treatment centers for mothers-to-be and newborn babies, sexually transmitted disease centers, a program for the provision of information on HIV/AIDS, and a one-stop crisis center for the management of survivors of violence against women and children.[15] Other treatments provided by ARROW aimed at promoting women's health include adopting the National Policy for Women's Health, which is a collaborative mechanism run jointly by government and nongovernmental agencies. This adds up to a significant level of service provision and should further improve the health facilities open to women.

Processes of migration and urbanization have significantly affected women's health. There has been a general migration from rural to urban areas as well as an overall increase in the number of working women. In order to curb the adverse effects of these changes, such as decline in the health status of people living in urban areas, the government is trying to provide low-cost housing for the urban poor, crèches at workplaces plus two months' leave for maternity and two weeks' leave for paternity. These policies are aimed at strengthening family institutions among Malaysians,[16] and the country is adopting a variety of strategies to reduce maternal morbidity and mortality. For example, a project called the *Safe Motherhood Initiative* has been implemented in selected districts with high maternal and prenatal mortality rates, in conjunction with other Asian countries such as Indonesia and Thailand. This is to help develop early warning devices to try and prevent prolonged labor that without intervention could otherwise turn into a life-threatening and obstructed labor.

SOCIAL POLICY AND CULTURAL MIX

Regarding the population of Malaysia, Malays and other Bumiputera groups make up 65% Chinese 26% Indians 8% and other unlisted ethnic groups comprise 1%. The country is officially Muslim, yet it has a wide variety of ethnic groups, and recognizing that religion and ethnicity are not necessarily the same, the interrelation between these cultural and ethnic groups forms an important part of Malaysian identity. During the British colonial period, Malays were the biggest population in Malaya, although in the Malay Peninsula and in some other areas, a mix of ethnic groups had long existed. Chinese and Indians migrated to Malaya in search of a livelihood, and this took place with the active encouragement of the British. Traditional beliefs and practices are nonetheless still strong among the Malays, and as Muslims, Malay people are accustomed to performing Islamic rituals, mastering doctrines and practicing sharia law. However, while Malaysian society is changing rapidly because of economic growth, interdependencies arising from a complex mix of cultural elements have prevented serious threats to national unity and political stability.

Although Malaysia is governed by a predominantly Malay Muslim government, there has been no attempt to oppress non-Muslims. The Malaysian government is tolerant and shows respect for religious observances of different religious groups. Although Islam is the official religion of Malaysia, other religion is allowed to be practiced. In Malaysia, Islam is the religion of only 60% of the people, and there is a general attitude of acceptance, tolerance and accommodation towards minorities on the part of the Muslim majority.

The progress of social policy in respect to Malaysian health care has been influenced by factors such as the involvement of government, equitable growth, levels of transparency and preference for moderation, as well as a degree of general and political consensus. The ruling party, the National Front (*Barisan Nasional*, previously known as the Alliance Party) gained support and confidence from the general population to administer the country from 1955 until the present day, which is one of the factors that has helped contribute to the success of social policy as a whole and to achieving a measure of economic balance.[18] Malaysia readily permits constructive criticism of its social policies, and non-governmental organizations, interest groups, and the public all have freedom to express their opinions. This should help to ensure social stability in the future, while at the same time making health improvement programs much easier to implement.

REFERENCES

1. *Institut Jantung Negara—National Heart Institute.* Information available from: www. ijn.com.my/new/index.php (accessed August 17, 2009).
2. United Nations. *Human Development Report 2006.* Available at: http://hdr.undp.org/ en/reports/global/hdr2006 (accessed August 17, 2009).
3. Economic Planning Unit: Prime Minister's Department. *Malaysia: 30 years of poverty reduction, growth and racial harmony. A case study report.* In: *Scaling Up Poverty Reduction: a global learning process and conference. A World Bank report.* Shanghai; May 2004.
4. Prime Minister's Department, Malaysia. Case study: *30 Years of poverty and reduction, growth and racial harmony.* Available at: http://unpan1.un.org/intradoc/ groups/public/documents/apcity/unpan021601.pdf www.hawaii.edu/hivandaids/ Malaysia__30_Years_of_Poverty_Reduction,_Growth_and_Racial_Harmony.pdf (accessed April 4, 2011).
5. Pillay S. Can we afford to fall sick? *Aliran Monthly.* 2005; **25**(4). Available at: http:// aliran.com/archives/monthly/2005a/4e.html (accessed September 19, 2009).
6. Economic Planning Unit, op. cit.
7. Malaysian Medical Association. *Health for All: reforming health care in Malaysia.* Selangor: Academe Art & Printing Services, MMA: 1999.
8. Chee HL. Ownership, control and contention: challenge for the future of healthcare in Malaysia. *Soc Sci Med.* 2008; **66**: 2145–56.
9. Barraclough S. The politics of privatization in the Malaysian health care system. *Journal of Contemporary Southeast Asia.* 2000; **22**: 340.
10. The World Health Report 2006: *Working together for health.* Geneva: WHO; 2006. Available at: www.who.int/whr/2006/en (accessed September 16, 2009).
11. Lim MK. Transforming Singapore healthcare: public-private partnership. *Ann Acad Med.* 2005: **34**(7): 461–7. Available at: www.annals.edu.sg/past.html (accessed September 16, 2009).
12. Asian-Pacific Resource and Research Centre for Women (ARROW). *See:* www.aworc. org/org/arrow/arrow.html (accessed July 29, 2009).
13. Morrow M, Barraclough S. Tobacco control and gender in Southeast Asia: (Part 1) Malaysia and the Phillipines. *Health Promotion International.* 2003; **18**(3): 255–64. Available at: http://heapro.oxfordjournals.org/cgi/content/full/18/3/255 (accessed 6 April 2011).
14. United Nations Economic and Social Commission for Western Asia. *Social Policies in Malaysia (3rd Report).* 2001. Available at: www.escwa.un.org/information/ publications.asp (accessed August 2, 2009).
15. Manaf RA, Shamsuddin K. Smoking among young urban Malaysian women and its risk factors. *Asia Pac J of Public Health.* 2008; **20**(3); 204–13.
16. ARROW, op. cit.
17. UN Economic and Social Commission for Western Asia. *Social Policies in Malaysia (4th Report).* 2003. Available at: www.escwa.un.org/information/publications/edit/ upload/ssd-03-1.pdf (accessed April 4, 2011).
18. Noor Sulastry Yurni Ahmad. The transformation in Malaysia's 12th general election: the end of National Front hegemony. *International Journal of Social Sciences* 2010; **9**(4); 69–80.

CHAPTER 8

Pharmaceutical industry, medicine and questions of ethics

a) Industry and the physician-investigator in the USA

Jaazzmina Hussain

BACKGROUND

The pharmaceutical industry is a major contributor of both financial and intellectual investment to research efforts aimed at advancing medical knowledge and capability. The number of physicians recruiting patients for enrollment into studies of novel therapies is rising, and in parallel, ethical issues around maintaining objectivity are becoming increasingly challenging.

In the USA, some regulatory mechanisms regarding conflicts of interest are at the federal level, and others take the form of voluntary codes of conduct, emanating from organizations such as the American Medical Association. These voluntary codes place reliance upon individual physician integrity to disclose ties with industry, but there have been occasions where financial ties between industry and the physician-investigator have not been properly disclosed. This can result in prejudicing the conduct of a clinical trial.[1]

CURRENT POLICIES AND CONSIDERATIONS

Federal governance of the physician-industry alliance relating to the advancement of medical knowledge and research comes from:
1 The Food and Drug Administration (FDA), which controls the marketing and distribution of novel therapies through enforcement of two laws: the *Code of*

Federal Regulations Title 21 Food and Drugs, and the *Food and Drug Administration Amendments Act (2007)*

2   The National Institutes of Health (NIH) and the Office for Human Research Protection (OHRP), which between them set national standards for ethical biomedical research

3   The Office of Research Integrity (ORI), which acts as a watchdog for research misconduct.

The majority of governance arrangements come from the lead professional bodies:

- The Pharmaceutical Researchers and Manufacturers of America (PhRMA), which represents its members and self-regulates most of the pharmaceutical companies, including global corporations such as Pfizer, Amgen-Wyeth and Merck
- The *American Medical Association* (AMA), which represents a proportion of doctors from all grades and all states across the USA; the AMA's opinions on ethical matters are powerful, influential and are often referred to by federal organizations on matters of health policy
- The American College of Physicians (ACP), which represents internal medicine physicians
- The Association of American Medical Colleges (AAMC), which represents medical schools of the USA and the academic medical centers where many physicians conduct their research.

In terms of the physician-investigator and the recruitment of subjects, a 2002 study placed the number of physicians involved in research at approximately 30 000. Around 60% of industry support for clinical trials goes to community-based studies, which take place in physicians' offices and clinics around the country.[2] Conflicts of interest essentially come about when a physician is paid to recruit patients and to do research on those for whom s/he has a primary duty of care. The combined roles of physician-healer and physician-investigator can give rise to concerns challenging the relationship that is predicated on trust between doctors and patients.

The professional medical associations prohibit the receipt of "finder's fees," which are payments made for referring patients to clinical trials, in an effort to try and prevent inappropriate patient recruitment in respect of lucrative remuneration packages offered by the pharmaceutical companies. However, the wording of policies about payments that physicians can accept is not explicit, using terms such as "reasonable remuneration," "recompense commensurate with effort," and "compensation for time and effort spent." These phrases occur in the policy literature but are clearly open to interpretation, especially since PhRMA agrees that it is acceptable to pay extra money to physicians where enrollment into a trial is particularly challenging.[3]

For example, if a family practitioner is asked to look through her patient lists and give all patients with hypertension the opportunity to be part of a trial testing a new medication, the doctor would be compensated for her time at the hourly rate she normally charges; however, how should effort be measured? If out of 100 hypertensive patients only three volunteer freely to participate in the trial, should the physician be paid more to persuade another 15 people to participate? Is such an arrangement rewarding a physician for placing her own interests above those of her patients?

The difficulty faced by pharmaceutical companies in this respect is how to ensure physicians recruit enough patients so that the trial has sufficient power, which necessarily means making it "worth the physician's while." Payments based on how many patients a physician enrolls are forbidden; however, a flat-rate payment for enrolling patients determined by the company and approved by institutional review boards (IRBs) prior to the recruitment process offers a workable solution. However, a problem arises regarding a "therapeutic misconception," which is the phenomenon that occurs despite a consent process explicitly stating that a trial, for example, of a novel antihypertensive drug, is not primarily intended to benefit that patient, yet the patient believes that the trial is part of his or her treatment and is therefore "in their best interests."[4] Broad distinctions between therapeutic and non-therapeutic trials may not be fully appreciated by patients. Ethically, it matters who is exposed to what risk and for whose benefit, and these matters are not simply points of theoretical interest.

The problem is made worse when the physician-investigator seeking to obtain the consent is also the patient-subject's primary physician. With lucrative compensations offered by the pharmaceutical company it is easy to see how physicians may seek to supplement their income by encouraging patients to enter a trial, emphasizing the positive aspects of participation. The AMA suggests that one way around this problem is to advise treating physicians not to be involved in the consent process.[5] However, therapeutic misconceptions may persist beyond the initial consent process, and were patients to experience minor but unpleasant side effects of the drug being trialed, they might refrain from exercising their right to withdraw from the trial for fear of disappointing the responsible physician or causing offense. In therapeutic trials this might be seen as "passing up the opportunity to receive a potentially life-saving drug," and physicians encouraging their patients to participate in trials must do so in ways that avoid limiting patient autonomy. As an ethical minimum, explanations must make it clear who stands to benefit (and in what way) from taking part in the process.

DISCLOSURE OF TRIAL SPONSORSHIP

In 2007, PhRMA companies invested $44.5 billion in the entire process of research and development of new drugs; by comparison, the NIH provided a total of $2.24

billion for the same year.[6] In order to improve transparency in the conduct of clinical trials, most pharmaceutical companies no longer research their own products; instead, work is outsourced to academic medical centers or to individual physicians working in private offices and clinics.

Codes issued by professional medical associations explicitly state that potential research subjects must be informed of the source of a trial's funding as part of the consent process. However, such a policy implies that patients have insight into industry involvements in medical research, and a 2006 survey of cancer patient opinions explicitly focused on these insights.[7] Out of the 253 patients interviewed, 90% expressed little or no concern over investigators' financial ties. Consistent with other trends in medicine, better educated patients were more likely to express concerns over financial ties that researchers had than less well educated patients. Nonetheless, this has little impact on the decision to participate, 70% declaring that they would participate regardless of any financial ties. When interviewed over what should be disclosed when and to whom, only 35% of subjects thought that patients should be more fully informed, and when asked about disclosure, 40% of subjects thought it was important to be informed about conflicts of interest but thought that an outside body should oversee these ties.

Though the results of this study suggest that patients are nonchalant over where the money for experimental treatments comes from, the study has its limitations. Firstly, the patient-subjects surveyed all had advanced cancers, and oncology is the key specialty in which clinical trial enrollment offers patients a way to access novel therapies that could extend life. It is natural that these patient-subjects would be more preoccupied with the fact that novel therapies might offer a chance of extended survival and be less worried about undisclosed finances ties. A comparison of opinion from patients affected by non-terminal illnesses would potentially provide valuable results, offering more meaningful insights into the nature of the problem. In an era of heightened awareness about physician ties with industry, such a study could even yield results that boosted public trust, which in turn could improve the rates of participation in clinical trials.

ENSURING OBJECTIVITY

The central issue of pharmaceutical industry involvement with medical research is in maintaining objectivity when funding for a trial comes from companies with a vested interest in the product. (For a comprehensive discussion of these issues, *see* Murray and Johnston, 2010.)[8] Pharmaceutical companies award research grants directly to individual physician-investigators who are often prominent figures in their chosen field. As NIH ethical principles suggest, research on human subjects is only ethical if the scientific methodology is sound. When conflict of interest interferes with the methodology or analysis of a trial, this challenges its ethical integrity.[9]

One way to mitigate against the corrosive effect of conflict of interest on scientific objectivity could be to ensure adequate public disclosure, and the new AAMC guidelines on maintaining objectivity and published in 2008 were issued just months before a major scandal broke about a physician-investigator in an academic medical center who failed to disclose the extent of his ties with industry. The system by which reports on conflicts of interest are made thereby came under close scrutiny following media revelations about substantial, undisclosed conflicts of interest. Unfortunately, as in the case involving Dr. Charles B. Nemeroff of Emory University, academic medical centers rely on physicians' integrity to report accurately on any financial ties that they have with industry, and in Nemeroff's case this did not happen.[10]

This evident failure of professional integrity sparked a congressional senator to propose a new law that would require pharmaceutical companies to reveal all payments made to physicians, enabling external bodies to be able to compare the payments made with those disclosed by the physicians. The *Physician Payments Sunshine Act* was eventually introduced into Congress in early 2009.[11] In matters of professional self-regulation, federal interventions of this kind are rare, and this would appear to be a direct response to the events just described.

Just as physician-investigators have a duty of care towards patient-subjects, pharmaceutical companies have an obligation to their shareholders, albeit of a different kind. With the average cost of research and development of novel therapies standing at around $800 million and taking between seven and 10 years to complete,[12] companies are unsurprisingly anxious to reduce costs and are committed to having products found to be effective and approved by the FDA as quickly as possible. Additionally, rising suspicions and increasing demands to have greater separation between physician-investigators and industry have given birth to a new enterprise in the form of Commercial Contract Research Organizations (CCROs).

CCROs, of which there are reported to be over 1,000 in the USA, are able to conduct any stage of the clinical trial process as well as compile study reports for publication.[13] Their services are in demand for reasons that include the ability of pharmaceutical companies to devolve much of the responsibility for conducting trials on to CCROs, thus allowing the original company to act only in the capacity of a sponsor and ostensibly removing any implied pressure on physicians towards bias in relation to trials.

Critics of CCRO involvement in clinical trials are skeptical of the purported degree of independence. If such companies exist solely to perform research, then positive results would confer repeat business, and so the objectivity of CCRO research cannot be guaranteed. As Lenzer writes, "You can ask a question which you know will give a favorable answer for the funder—and not ask other questions."[14] Reliance is placed in IRBs to oversee these trials, making questions about their independence critical, although this is not something that can be evaluated here. A number of CCROs maintain academic connections through awarding consultancy contracts and royalties. These academic centers provide credibility that eminent researchers bring to the CCROs, making it difficult to distinguish this type of situation from ones in which pharmaceutical companies make grants directly to an individual.

REMUNERATION OF PHYSICIAN-INVESTIGATORS

The work and effort that many physician-investigators put into the conduct of scientifically (and ethically) sound research cannot be denied, and that they should be paid fairly for what they contribute is without question. Professional institutional policies explicitly state that physicians must only accept payment for work they have done, and the amount accepted must be commensurate with the levels of service provided. There must also be a written contract between the physician and the pharmaceutical company enumerating the services for which they are being paid.[15] These arrangements reflect the current standard.

Although ethical considerations surrounding gifts to physicians are outside of the scope of this chapter, nevertheless, it is important to consider the acceptability of the inclusion of additional research grants, consultancy arrangements, speaker fees and royalties into remuneration packages called "salary." For example, arrangements that include extra grants for clinical or laboratory equipment could also be construed as gifts to encourage overall results that would please a sponsor. The apparent acceptability of such arrangements contrasts with a PhRMA decision to prohibit company representatives from providing physicians with low-value gifts such as pens, notepaper and mugs that supposedly influence physicians' habits when prescribing.

At face value, this does seem inconsistent from a policy point of view in that there can be substantial amounts of money involved in the compensation that physician-investigators receive for performing trials and speaking about post-trial successes. Although payment for services rendered should not be tied to the outcome of a trial, it stands to reason that physicians know they are unlikely to be offered a several thousand-dollar contract to lecture about a drug that fails.

COMMUNICATING RESULTS

A number of issues arise when considering the conduct of physician-investigators in communicating trial results. Firstly, there is the problem of bias, whereby failure to report serious adverse reactions to a drug could reduce its marketability, and secondly, there is the question of bias in altering the fidelity and integrity of publication content. Thirdly, there are difficulties with disclosing conflicts of interest at the point of publication and how this can affect the way in which a paper is read. (The Vioxx scandal that came to light in 2007 is an example of how selective reporting of clinical trial data can affect patient care.)[16]

On occasions, adverse effects only come to light after a trial has finished, and a the physician-investigator plays a role in bringing these adverse events to light. A balance has to be struck between protecting patients from harm by thorough investigation, and the timely release of products onto the market. This balance may be achieved by conducting mandatory post-marketing studies, which is a strategy the FDA has considered. Such a scheme could be beneficial in obtaining data on efficacy as well as safety; however, there could be difficulties in preventing such studies from becoming "seeding trials," i.e. trials whose purpose is to generate increases in prescriptions for a particular drug. Conversely, a case could be made asking "how can data on safety and efficacy be obtained without adequate usage?," and this counter-argument has some validity.[17]

The concern that reports of industry-funded trials automatically introduce bias in favor of a product being studied regardless of the results is not without foundation. A 2006 study of concordance between financial ties and industry support in meta-analysis of anti-hypertensive drugs found that although sponsorship from drug companies was not associated with positive results, it did not rule out the possibility of an association between industry funding and positive reports.[18]

Physicians seem to be aware of the possibility that industry-sponsored research is inherently biased, and a small 2004 study looked at whether details of disclosure did affect the credibility of a study to an audience of doctors.[19] It found that the sample paper which disclosed a financial tie scored lower in areas of importance, relevance, validity and believability than the sample paper, for which no financial interests had been declared. Although the sample size was small and the subjects were attuned to the purpose of the study, such results are no less interesting and provide an insight into why some physicians seek to conceal or downplay their connections with industry.

GHOSTWRITING

On the subject of authorship, ghost-writing of scientific articles by authors paid by the pharmaceutical industry is sometimes seen as a less prominent issue by those calling for transparency in the physician-industry alliance. Nevertheless, estimates that at least 50% of all papers on treatments published in the *British Medical Journal*, *The Lancet* and *The New England Journal of Medicine* having been written by an unacknowledged source suggest that ghostwriting needs to be openly discussed.[20]

There are legitimate concerns over the true independence of the ghostwriter; firstly, a ghostwriter is under contract with a pharmaceutical company, just the same as the physician-investigator; secondly, if he or she is a permanent employee, that person clearly has an allegiance to the employer, leaving open the possibility of bias in the analysis and presentation of data. Ethically, ghostwriters must adopt a "corporeal form" and take their place amongst the credited authors, thus disclosing any competing interests and removing their status as a mere "ghost."[21] Better still, they should not be employed at all. Additionally, named authors must have made a substantial contribution to the manuscript and not solely attached their name to a manuscript written by someone else.

CONCLUSION

A trend towards aggressively managing conflicts of interest between physician-investigators and pharmaceutical companies has emerged. This is in response to increased public mistrust of the effect this relationship has on scientific integrity. But on the other hand, there are a growing number of professionals who believe the "hunt" has gone far enough. There is a growing but still limited body of evidence to suggest that conflicts of interest contribute to the under-reporting of negative effects and adverse outcomes of clinical trials,[22] even though penalties for research misconduct for pharmaceutical companies are significant. If conflicts of interest cannot be controlled, even with federal policing, it must ultimately be the responsibility of individual physicians and their academic institutions to safeguard scientific integrity by developing methods for policing inherent conflicts of interest between physician-investigators and the pharmaceutical industry.

REFERENCES

1. Ross J, Hill K, Egilman D, *et al*. Guest authorship and ghostwriting in publications related to rofecoxib: a case study of industry documents from rofecoxib litigation. *JAMA*. 2008; **299**: 1800–12.
2. Morin K, Rakatansky H, Riddick Jnr F, *et al*. Managing conflicts of interest in the conduct of clinical trials. *JAMA*. 2002; **287**: 78–84.
3. Pharmaceutical Manufacturers and Researchers of America. *Principles on conduct of clinical trials and the communication of results*. Washington, DC: PhRMA; 2004.
4. Ross, op. cit.
5. American Medical Association. *Code of Medical Ethics*. Available at: www.ama-assn.org/ama/pub/physician-resources/medical-ethics/code-medical-ethics.shtml (accessed September 20, 2009).
6. Pharmaceutical Manufacturers and Researchers of America. *Annual Report*. PhRMA; 2008.
7. Hampson L, Agrawal M, Joffe S, *et al*. Patients' views on financial conflicts of interest in cancer research trials. *NEJM*. 2006; **355**: 2330–7. Available at: http://content.nejm.org/cgi/reprint/355/22/2330.pdf (accessed September 20, 2009).
8. Murray TH, Johnston J, editors. *Trust and Integrity in Biomedical Research*. Maryland, USA: The Johns Hopkins University Press; 2010.
9. National Institutes of Health. *Ethics in Clinical Research*. Available at: http://clinical-research.nih.gov/ethics_guides.html (accessed September 20, 2009).
10. Harris G. Top psychiatrist did not report drug makers' pay. *New York Times*, October 3, 2008. Available at: www.nytimes.com/2008/10/04/health/policy/04drug.html?pagewanted=1&_r=1&sq=nemeroff&st=cse&scp=1 (accessed September 20, 2009).

11. U.S. Congress Track, S.301. 111th Congress. *Physician Payments Sunshine Act 2009.* Available at: www.govtrack.us/congress/bill.xpd?bill=s111-301 (accessed September 19, 2009).
12. Hampson, op. cit.
13. Lenzer J. Truly independent research? *BMJ.* 2008; **337**: 602–7.
14. Ibid.
15. Ross, op. cit.
16. Krumholz H, Ross J, Pressler A, *et al.* What have we learned from Vioxx®? *BMJ.* 2007; **334**: 120–3.
17. Psaty B, Rennie B. Clinical trial investigators and their prescribing patterns: another dimension to the relationship between physician investigators and the pharmaceutical industry. *JAMA.* 2006; **295**(23): 2787–90.
18. Yank V, Rennie D, Bero L. Financial ties and concordance between results and conclusions in meta-analyses: retrospective cohort study. *BMJ.* 2007; **335**: 1202–5.
19. Schroter S, Morris J, Chaudhry S, *et al.* Does the type of competing interest statement affect readers' perceptions of the credibility of research? *BMJ.* 2004; **328**: 742–3.
20. Dawes K. Ghost-writers need to be more visible. *BMJ.* 2007; **334**: 208.
21. Ibid.
22. Stossel T. Has the hunt for conflicts of interest gone too far? Yes. *BMJ.* 2008; **336**: 476.

b) Postgraduate medical education in the USA

Caroline Broughton

BACKGROUND

In the USA, continuing medical education (CME) for physicians is essential in order for them to keep their knowledge and skills up to date and maintain their license to practice. On account of the high costs involved, it is difficult for CME events to be put on without industry income; however, industry sponsorship of CME leads to conflicts of interest concerning how educational materials related to that corporation's products are presented, i.e. how they are presented in an unbiased manner. Since the education the physician receives is then utilized in patient care activities, the ethical question is whether industry support for CME unduly influences physician behavior in favor of the sponsoring corporation. Concerns have been raised both at the federal and professional levels that these conflicts of interest could compromise patient care. The notion currently being explored is that conflicts of interest cannot be excluded while the pharmaceutical industry has such a significant presence within the medical profession, and that more formal regulation and management of conflicts may be a matter of necessity. Both pharmaceutical companies and the medical profession need to take responsibility for any conflicts that are created, and both parties need to be honest in disclosing industry funding, with information made readily available to patients and to government.

CME consists of a variety of educational activities that serve to maintain and expand the skills, knowledge and professionalism of a physician with regard to service provision for patients and the general public.[1] In the USA, CME requirements for licensure (registration) and re-licensure vary depending on the state in which the physician works. Besides the pharmaceutical industry, funding for CME comes from government as well as other private sources. The Accreditation Council for Continuing Medical Education (ACCME) *Annual Data Report* states that total income for CME in 2007 was just over $2.5 billion, and of that, $1.2 billion came from commercial support, with a further $274 million coming from advertising and exhibits. These are substantial sums, with over half of the total CME income in 2007 coming from industry sources.[2] The moral question that needs to be asked is: "What is expected in return?"—or to put it more directly, is primary motivation behind this support to accrue increased sales, and if so, what is the price of this support?

ACCME is an independent body that recognizes and accredits organizations and institutions that offer CME, and in order for educational programs to be accredited they must meet ACCME Standards of Commercial Support in order to ensure a measure of independence from commercial interest. The American Medical Association (AMA) *Code of Ethics* states that as physicians have a fiduciary relationship with their patients it is essential for them to understand notions of professionalism, including conflicts of interest, for physicians to avoid compromising patient care.[3]

Further guidelines on conflict of interest clearly state that there are no circumstances under which a physician's financial interests can override concern for the welfare of patients, and if conflicts arise that potentially compromise patient care, then the best interests of patients must be the priority.[4] While practice standards are regulated at the state level, it is nominally the AMA that sets standards for the medical profession. However, it is not a regulatory body and membership is entirely voluntary; of the 900 000 practicing physicians in the US only around 245 000 are members of the AMA, and 30% of this figure includes medical students and residents. Therefore, it does not speak for the profession as a whole.

There is evidence suggesting that physicians are generally unaware of the bias created by receiving gifts from industry and reluctant to see that accepting a gift could be perceived as unethical.[5] Physicians unintentionally do what is in their own best interests, and can have difficulty taking a neutral perspective when they have a personal interest in an event. These concerns were heightened in 2007 when the Attorney General of Vermont reported that US psychiatrists received more money from consulting arrangements with pharmaceutical companies (including payment for presenting at CME events) than doctors in any other specialty.[6] There is widespread concern that this type of payment creates bias and influences the prescribing practice of physicians, and drug marketing disclosures in Vermont show payments to physician-prescribers between July 2007 and 2008 amounting to $3 million,[7] which is no trivial amount considering that Vermont is not a large state. In addition, data from Minnesota shows that psychiatrists who received in excess of $5,000 from pharmaceutical companies that produce newer generation antipsychotic drugs were three times more likely to write off-label, i.e. scripts not explicitly approved by the Food and Drug Administration for using that class of drug.[8]

INTERACTIONS WITH HEALTH CARE PROFESSIONALS

PhRMA, the association representing research-based pharmaceutical and biotechnology companies, issued a revised *Code on Interactions with Health care Professionals* in 2008, reflecting concerns that their members' interactions with health care professionals could be perceived as inappropriate by patients and by the public more generally. The code is designed to reinforce all industry interactions with medical professionals to benefit patients and professional practice as a whole.[9]

Revisions to the updated code include the following:

1 There is a complete ban on all company-branded, non-educational items, such as pens and mugs, which were previously freely available at CME events, since there is recognition that these items may be perceived to create bias.

2 Companies should separate their grant-making department from sales and marketing, and objective criteria should be applied when deciding which genuinely educational CME events to support.
3 Companies should ensure that their representatives are appropriately trained regarding laws and regulations on conflicts of interest about relationships between industry and the profession.
4 Companies should audit their representatives on a regular basis and take appropriate action if they fail to comply with current standards.

Companies who abide by the Code can make their intentions clear via a publicly accessible website. Chief Executive Officers must certify each year that their companies are still compliant. (At the time of this writing, the names of 48 pharmaceutical companies have appeared on the PhRMA website stating their intention to comply with the new Code.)

COMPLIANCE PROGRAM GUIDANCE
FOR PHARMACEUTICAL MANUFACTURERS

The Office of Inspector General (OIG) in the US Department of Health and Human Services issued guidelines in 2003 questioning the legality of the interactions between the pharmaceutical industry and health care providers. The OIG wanted to address aspects of physician industry relationships, including industry funding of educational events and the provision of "gifts," the concern being that while such interactions are not illegal, there is scope for abuse of "anti-kickback" laws.[10] Government health care programs needed to have protection from abuses that could potentially harm patients if there is evidence that industry money unduly influences doctors.

At the present time, OIG guidelines are supportive of PhRMA recommendations, stating that gifts of any value have the potential to invoke anti-kickback law if there is any intention to promote business for the pharmaceutical companies in question.[11] The hope is that compliance with the PhRMA code should reduce the risk of fraud and abuse. OIG guidelines, however, do not offer advice on monitoring exchanges between the industry and the professionals, and although the issue is addressed in the 2009 PhRMA code, this is an area that could potentially benefit from additional federal regulation.

The Council on Ethical and Judicial Affairs (CEJA) of the AMA published a report in May 2009 titled *Financial Relationships with Industry in Continuing Medical Education*, which put forward suggestions to formally address these conflicts of interest.[12] Three options were presented. Firstly, the problem of bias could be avoided by not permitting conditions that may give rise to it; secondly, strategies could be implemented to mitigate bias or influence, and thirdly, a combination of both, which might offer the best solution. It concluded by making the following recommendations based on the premise that it is the responsibility of the physician to actively seek CME events that are ethically preferable or ethically permissible:

Preferred events include those where the funding received has no direct influence on the clinical recommendations.

Permissible events include those where industry funding has a more direct impact but which are adequately disclosed.[13]

CONCLUSION

The issue of conflicts of interest will always remain a problem while the pharmaceutical industry continues to provide a significant amount of financial support for continuing medical education. In order to maintain the moral integrity of the profession and maintain public trust, industry and the medical profession need to manage these conflicts through enforceable regulation at federal or state level and voluntary codes of conduct through professional organizations. Most current policies are based on guidelines and depend on the honesty and integrity of individual physicians to be honest about their industry ties, and to be responsible when attending CME events deemed *"ethically preferable."* There is greater transparency now than before as regards these matters, but how effective voluntary codes prove in regulating practice is something that remains to be seen.

REFERENCES

1. American Medical Association. *Be Recognized ... for your commitment to patient care through continuing medical education.* AMA information on CME. Available at: www.ama-assn.org/ama1/pub/upload/mm/455/praapplication.pdf (accessed September 19, 2009).
2. The Accreditation Council for Continuing Medical Education. *Annual Report Data, 2007.* Available at: www.accme.org/dir_docs/doc_upload/207fa8e2-bdbe-47f8-9b65-52477f9faade_uploaddocument.pdf (accessed September 19, 2009).
3. American Medical Association. *Code of Medical Ethics, 2001.* Available at: www.ama-assn.org/ama/pub/physician-resources/medical-ethics/code-medical-ethics/principles-medical-ethics.shtml (accessed September 19, 2009).
4. American Medical Association. *Opinion 8.03—Conflicts of Interest.* Guidelines, 1994. Available at: www.ama-assn.org/ama/pub/physician-resources/medical-ethics/code-medical-ethics/opinion803.shtml (accessed September 19, 2009).
5. Dana J, Loewenstein G. A social science perspective on gifts to physicians from industry. *JAMA.* 2003; **290**(2): 252–5.
6. Office of the Attorney General of Vermont (William H Sorrell). *Pharmaceutical Marketing Disclosures Report, 2007.* Available at: www.atg.state.vt.us/issues/pharmaceutical-manufacturer-payment-disclosure/pharmaceutical-marketing-disclosures-reports.php (accessed October 2, 2009).
7. Office of the Attorney General of Vermont. *Disclosures of Marketing Expenditures for Prescription Drugs, Biological Products and Medical Devices.* Available at: www.atg.

state.vt.us/issues/pharmaceutical-manufacturer-payment-disclosure.php (accessed October 2, 2009).

8. Harris G, Carey B, Roberts J. Psychiatrists, children and drug industry's role. *New York Times*. May 10, 2008. Available at: www.nytimes.com/2007/05/10/health/10psyche. html?scp=1&sq=Psychiatrists%2C+children+and+drug+industry%92s+role&st=nyt (accessed September 20, 2009).

9. PhRMA. *PhRMA Code on interactions with healthcare professionals*. Washington, DC. 2008 (effective January 2009). Available at: www.phrma.org/sites/default/files/369/ phrma_marketing_code_2008-1.pdf www.phrma.org/option,com_pressreleases/ Itemid,41 (accessed April 4, 2011).

10. Chimonas S, Rothman DJ. New federal guidelines for physician-pharmaceutical industry relations: the politics of policy formation. *Health Affairs*. 2005; **24**(4): 949–60.

11. US Government Office of Public Affairs. *Federal Anti-kickback Law and Regulatory Safe Harbors*. Fact sheet (1999). Available at: http://oig.hhs.gov/fraud/docs/safeharbor-regulations/safefs.htm (accessed September 19, 2009).

12. American Medical Association. *Council on Ethical and Judicial Affairs Report 1-A-09*. Available at: www.ama-assn.org/ama1/pub/upload/mm/475/ceja01a09.pdf (accessed September 19, 2009).

13. Ibid.

CHAPTER 9

Geneva to Guantanamo and the ethics of interrogation

Maya Prabhu

INTRODUCTION

The US military's detention facility at Guantanamo Bay in Cuba (hereinafter "Guantanamo") has been the subject of considerable controversy since it was reopened in 2002. It was previously a detention center for Haitian refugees, and Guantanamo really only became prominent in the aftermath of the terrorist atrocities in September 2001 and the invasion of Iraq in 2003. Prisoners captured in the so-called "War on Terror" were taken there on the advice of the US Justice Department, which was seeking a location suited to its purposes outside US legal jurisdiction. Much of the controversy centered on the use of Guantanamo to hold non-US citizens believed to be threats for indefinite periods of time. Though military authorities at the Pentagon have been obscure about details of the detainees held there, it is believed that a total of 780 individuals have passed through the facility.[1,2]

Almost immediately after Guantanamo's reopening, a tsunami of sources, including investigative journalists, non-governmental organizations and the International Committee of the Red Cross (ICRC), started to raise concerns that detainees were being subjected to torture and a variety of degrading practices. These practices were said to include sleep deprivation, prolonged isolation, painful body positions, sensory deprivation, feigned suffocation, beatings, temperature extremes and waterboarding; other stress-inducing tactics included sexual provocation, forced grooming and displays of contempt for Islamic symbols.[3] These concerns have been steadily confirmed by a large number of US government documents that were obtained by the American Civil Liberties Union under the US Freedom of Information Act.[4] This gave rise to serious concerns about the way in which long-established ethical and legal frameworks were being set aside in the interests of "national security."

Some of the most bruising criticism of Guantanamo was directed at health professionals and the apparent erosion of military medical ethics and practices being carried out in the name of "intelligence gathering." Furthermore, sources that documented torture indicated that health professionals—psychiatrists, psychologists and other medical personnel—were both tacitly and actively involved with detainee mistreatment. Lapses ranged from not maintaining medical records to failing to conduct medical examinations and provide proper care, terminating detainee hunger strikes, and falsifying medical records and death certificates. Perhaps the most egregious of all was the use of medical information and medical personnel to design and implement psychologically and physically coercive experiences. In its assessment of Guantanamo interrogations, the ICRC concluded that "*[health personnel's] primary purpose appears to have been to serve the interrogation process, and not the patient. In so doing the health personnel have condoned and participated in ill-treatment,*" ill-treatment which constituted a "*gross breach of medical ethics and, in some cases, amounted to participation in torture…*"[5] In sum, how detainees at Guantanamo were treated is something that warrants close scrutiny.

DOCTORS' INVOLVEMENT WITH DETAINEE 063 (*SEE* BOX 1)

There is sizeable literature describing the involvement of medical military personnel in interrogations at Guantanamo.[6a,b,c,d,e] For a vivid explication of medical involvement, readers are invited to review the interrogation logs of Detainee 063, Mohammed al-Qahtani, known as the 20th hijacker. The full logs were first obtained by *TIME* magazine reporters in 2005, and they have been analyzed extensively by numerous writers and medical and legal experts.[7a,b,c] For over 50 days, al-Qahtani was questioned for 18 hours a day, threatened with dogs, taunted by female interrogators, subjected to temperature extremes and loud sounds (including the music of Christina Aguilera) and forced to wear women's undergarments, all while being allowed only four hours of sleep a night.

As the excerpts in Box 1 illustrate, contrary to the military's early denials of medical involvement, health professionals were directly involved in al-Qahtani's treatment. During periods of questioning, al-Qahtani was assessed and hospitalized for hypothermia, treated for dehydration, prescribed enemas for constipation, and assessed for swollen feet. Blood was taken and analyzed, electrolytes were monitored and an ultrasound performed to rule out the possibility of a blood clot. An observing psychologist advised interrogators how to disorient and humiliate the detainee, and psychological themes of "guilt/sin" and "futility" were used in conjunction with other degrading techniques to assert interrogators' control over the prisoner.

Though the al-Qahtani interrogation is the only extensive interrogation publicly available at the time of writing, the techniques used are consistent with reports of other detainees and high-level internal memoranda outlining interrogation methods.[8] It is reasonable to extrapolate from al-Qahtani's experience and apply it to other detainees, and if anything, recent evidence indicates that interrogations have become more brutal, consisting of *"unauthorized, improvised, inhumane and undocumented"* methods such as threatening suspects with a gun and a power drill, threatening to sexually abuse a detainee's mother, and applying pressure to a carotid artery until the detainee loses consciousness.[9] Even without knowledge of ethical and legal codes that apply to medicine, these accounts are harrowing, and it is hard to imagine anything more unethical or distasteful in terms of actions carried out by qualified health professionals.

EXISTING LEGAL AND ETHICAL FRAMEWORKS

The transcripts are shocking and speak badly of US government-sponsored standards of interrogation, but they also beg the question of how health professionals became such willing accomplices. Until this time, international law and codes of ethics devised after the Nuremberg trials of 1948 had been thought sufficient to inhibit doctors from taking part in this kind of abuse. The US government signed and enacted numerous international declarations and conventions prohibiting torture and the abuse of human rights, including:

- The UN Convention against Torture and Other Cruel, Inhuman, or Degrading Treatment or Punishment, which defines "torture" as "any act by which severe pain or suffering, whether physical or mental, is intentionally inflicted on a person for such purposes as obtaining from him or a third person information or a confession, ... at the instigation of ... a public official"[10]
- The UN Universal Declaration of Human Rights, which stipulates that "No one shall be subjected to torture or cruel, inhumane or degrading treatment or punishment"[11]
- The Geneva Convention Common Article Three, relative to the Treatment of Prisoners of War, which lists among other protections that "Persons ... placed *hors de combat* by ... detention shall in all circumstances be treated humanely; ... to this end the following acts are and shall remain prohibited at any time and in any place whatsoever [to include] outrages upon personal dignity, [and] in particular, humiliating and degrading treatment; ... no physical or mental torture, nor any other form of coercion, may be inflicted on prisoners of war to secure from them information of any kind whatever. Prisoners of war who refuse to answer may not be threatened, insulted, or exposed to any unpleasant or disadvantageous treatment of any kind"[12]
- UN Body of Principles for the Protection of All Persons under Any Form of Detention or Imprisonment, and UN Standard Minimum Rules for the Treatment of Prisoners.[13]

Additionally, domestic US military internment and interrogation policies collectively bar US armed forces from practicing torture or degrading treatments of all persons.[14] The US Army Field Manual in particular includes specific prohibitions, including forced nudity, forced sexual acts, hooding, beating, shocking, burning, waterboarding, hypothermia, mock executions and the use of dogs—all of which have come to light at Guantanamo.

Professional codes of ethics that apply to the conduct of health professionals routinely ground the individual doctor-patient relationship on principles of autonomy, beneficence and justice, and the 1975 World Medical Association (WMA) Declaration of Tokyo provides "Guidelines for Physicians Concerning Torture and other Cruel, Inhuman or Degrading Treatment or Punishment in Relation to Detention and Imprisonment." It states that in "all cases at all times, physician(s) shall not countenance, condone or participate in torture or any other form of abuse; nor use nor allow to be used [their] medical knowledge or skills, or health information to aid interrogation in any way; nor be present during any procedure during which torture or any other forms of cruel, inhuman or degrading treatment is used or threatened."[15]

There are no special ethical codes for active-duty military physicians, although the "dual loyalty" dilemma has long been recognized.[16] Dual loyalty, or the concept that physicians have obligations to a patient and a third party, or a patient and a broader social purpose, is not unknown to civilian physicians. For example, it could include mandatory reporting of child abuse or sharing physical exam results with an insurance company. However, military personnel face particular dilemmas when the social purpose is "national security" and when the "third party" consists of military commanders.

Notwithstanding such complexities, there is a consensus that military health personnel are bound by the same medical ethics obligations as civilians.[17a,b,c] Moreover, unlike civilians, military health personnel explicitly take an oath to the Constitution, including the Fifth, Eighth and Fourteenth Amendments, which collectively prohibit torture.[18] Additionally, unique to the military medical experience are staffing detention facilities where the historic rule is that "soldiers, POWs and detainees are entitled to the same [professional] standard of care ..."[19,20] The extraordinary nature of events at Guantanamo is indicated by letters sent to both Congress and the President by retired senior officers, who describe the abuse of prisoners as anathema to the military's historic principles, and "beyond *what was allowed by the Army Field Manual.*"[21]

CULTURAL CHANGES POST-9/11

Tragically, there is a long history of physician involvement in torture and abuse, which during the 20th century included Nazi death camps and apartheid-era South Africa.[22a,b,c,d] Perhaps it ought not be shocking that physicians, psychologists and other health care workers at Guantanamo became ensnared in military interrogations and mistreatment. However, it must be asked whether ethical and cultural

frameworks changed after 9/11 in ways that facilitated the use of health professionals in situations involving interrogation.

In answer to that question, there can be little doubt that space for torture was
created by White House Counsel, as evidenced by Department of Justice memos
that began in 2002.[23] These legal opinions expressly removed the protection of the
Geneva Conventions from suspected War on Terror captives on the grounds that the
Taliban violated the rules of the Geneva Conventions by *"using civilians as human
shields,"* amongst other concerns.[24] Secondly, these documents redefined torture
downward—distinguishing it from cruel, inhuman or degrading treatment—and
permitting it in US centers.

Torture was then identified as physical pain inflicted *"of an intensity that accom-
panies serious physical injury such as death or organ failure."* Mental torture could only
be so described if it produced *"lasting psychological harm."* A subsequent Presidential
Executive Order reaffirmed this rejection of Geneva Convention guidelines on interrogations, even as it insisted that *"the United States Armed Forces shall continue to treat
detainees humanely and, to the extent appropriate and consistent with military necessity, in
a manner consistent with the principles of Geneva."*[25,26]

Though most of these legal stances have since been repudiated by the US administration (for example, in 2006 the US Supreme Court rejected President Bush's position that the Geneva Conventions did not apply to the conflict with al-Qaeda),[27] in
the early phase of the War on Terror, they created a legal vacuum that drew health
professionals into the process of gathering intelligence. Psychiatrists and psychologists in particular were recruited on Behavioral Science Consultation Teams (BSCT).
BSCT members' primary task was to engineer the camp experiences of "priority"
detainees to make interrogations more fruitful. Though they had no specific training in behavioral analysis, BSCT consultants prepared psychological profiles for
use by interrogators; they sat in on some interrogations and observed others from
behind one-way mirrors, offering feedback to the interrogators.

Eventually, Guantanamo became known as a "battle lab for new interrogation
techniques," techniques that were applied at military prisons in Iraq and Afghanistan
and at CIA detention centers.[28] As part of this interrogation, "lab" elements from the
Survival, Evasion, Resistance and Escape (SERE) program, taught at Fort Bragg and
developed by US psychologists to train US troops to resist torture, were "reverse
engineered" at Guantanamo Bay to create additionally coercive techniques against
detainees. Despite objections from Fort Bragg instructors as well as other military
personnel about applying SERE out of context[29] SERE tactics were nonetheless used
extensively.

LESSONS TO BE LEARNED

At a time when the military was under pressure to do everything possible to prevent
further terrorist attacks, it is easy to imagine the pressure on military personnel at

Guantanamo Bay to obtain good intelligence. It is equally easy to see how insidious Justice and Defense memos were creating an ethos in which professional medical obligations were subordinated to anxieties about collective survival and other military priorities.[30] The American Psychological Association's Ethics Task Force on National Security Interrogations went so far as to make its ethics policy conform with Pentagon guidelines governing psychologists' participation in interrogations—a position that led to calls for an independent investigation of the American Psychological Association (APA). The APA conducted a referendum and subsequently banned psychologists from facilities that violate US and international human rights law.[31] Added to the sense of urgency was the possibility that, because terrorism had been inextricably linked to people from Middle Eastern and Muslim backgrounds, it generated a type of extreme prejudice that somehow gave moral license to torturers.[32] As a result, human rights were allowed to be overlooked and violated solely in order to elicit information.

The real issue is not whether health professionals should return to historic standards of conduct, but how to ensure that professional ethics, medical codes, and international and domestic laws never again become subordinate to unilateral reinterpretation of legal doctrine. There is a tendency amongst physicians to be deferential towards legal and military authority, especially in situations of apparent urgency, rather than to trust moral intuition, such that some things are seen as being non-negotiable. Principles of medical ethics oppose any non-therapeutic interventions that take place in brutalizing scenarios such as those seen at Guantanamo. It is unfortunate that in the period after 9/11 a debate opened up, not about how medical personnel can resist pressures to cede their social obligations, but about how they should participate in torture as part of their social responsibilities. Though the medical community may feel helpless in the face of these security pressures, in fact, their socially validated role to respect the dignity of all individuals gives it tremendous moral leverage. Conversely, complicity with abuses of power and authority undermines medical professional credibility, both in peacetime and during war.

There were a variety of proposed responses to the details of medical involvement that came to light. In terms of legislative interventions, Senator John McCain, himself a survivor of torture, piloted legislation through the US Senate requiring detainees, wherever held, to be treated humanely. This principle is now enshrined in the Detainee Treatment Act of 2005,[33] the provisions of which are being used as the basis for action in a US Federal Court by lawyers acting on behalf of four hunger strikers at Guantanamo Bay. In a similar vein, the AMA House of Delegates adopted a new ethics policy on the participation of physicians in interrogations in 2006. This new policy prohibits physicians' involvement on BSCTs,[34] and the AMA has reiterated its support for international ethics codes and humanitarian law. Many have called for legal and licensing repercussions for physicians known to have participated in Guantanamo interrogations. For example, formal complaints with the state medical boards of Georgia and California have been lodged against the former hospital commander at Guantanamo Bay, John Edmondson, alleging that he violated the Declarations of Tokyo and Malta, to which the AMA is a signatory. Although the California Board has declined jurisdiction over the matter, the Georgia complaint is still pending and an appeal is likely in California. Finally, numerous organizations have suggested that independent commissions or investigations should be established to investigate how military health personnel were co-opted into coercive interrogation practices. One creative suggestion is that Guantanamo should be converted into a biomedical research institute dedicated to combating diseases of poverty, to serve as a kind of atonement for what happened.[35]

Above all, it seems clear that the Department of Defense needs to end and repudiate its practices of employing medical professional personnel in interrogations, and to affirm that military physicians should not compromise medical ethics when performing military duty in the future.[36] Unequivocal guidance is necessary in order for physicians to be able to give patients' needs the highest priority without fear of legal or military reprimand. In 2002, if a clear rule had been in existence against participation, acknowledging military health providers' multiple roles, it is hard to see how anyone would have felt able to participate in interrogation stressor techniques that were employed at Guantanamo.

While many have said it is largely incumbent upon the medical community to sustain resistance against the erosion of its ethical principles, Xenakis, a retired Brigadier-General and psychiatrist, may be right in saying that failings of medical personnel at Guantanamo Bay ultimately rest with senior military and medical leadership. Commanders are ultimately responsible for the ethical and moral climate within their units.[37] Formal recognition by the high-level military that what medical professionals did was wrong both legally and morally, not just tactically, would be the best way to reinvigorate respect for human rights, humanitarian law and medical ethics. Absent a *mea culpa* response, military and medical commitment to ethics and law continues to be fragile, meaning that it would not be impossible for them to be subverted again the future.

Box 1: Interrogation log of detainee 063[38]

December 4, 2002

1300: Detainee complained of dizziness. His vital signs were checked. Christina Aguilera's music was played.

1410: Vital signs were checked.

1540: Detainee refused water. Interrogation session now focused on "circumstantial evidence."

1740: Doctor checked patients' vital signs. Detainee determined to be dehydrated. Doctor drew blood to check kidney function.

1800: Medic inserted two IV tubes. Detainee complained about the presence and touch of a female, attempted to get out of seat and restraints.

1900: Detainee refused water and food.

2200: Detainee had been silent for two hours.

2300: Detainee exercised to reduce swelling in hands and feet.

December 5, 2002

0025: Detainee complained of tiredness. Detainee's hands were strung above head to reduce swelling from earlier IV. Detainee made to stand to improve circulation. Detainee refused water…

Day 15—December 7, 2002

001: Detainee made to stand for the National Anthem … Detainee taken to porch where he could see foraging banana rats …

0350: Vitals show dehydration is beginning. Detainee was given an IV by corpsman. Detainee was told we would not allow him to die …

1100: Schedule is given to MPs to … keep music playing to prevent detainee from sleeping … detainee's pulse is unusually slow … heartbeat is regular but very slow—35 bpm. Decision is made to take detainee to GTMO hospital to perform a CT scan of the detainee's brain to see if there are any irregularities …

2330: Doctors review scan and do not find any conclusive evidence of any conditions.

Day 18—December 10, 2002

001: Lead established control over detainee by instructing him not to speak and enforcing by playing loud music and yelling …

1930: Medical representative weighed detainee and logged detainee's weight at 119 pounds …

2230: Detainee urinated on himself as he was being taken to latrine.

December 13, 2002

0001: Detainee's hands were cuffed at his sides to prevent him from conducting his prayer ritual …

0025: Lead taped picture of [WTC] 3-year-old victim over detainee's heart … Control drips a few drops of water on detainee's head to keep him awake. Detainee struggles when the water is dropped on his head …

0120: Interrogators take a break and detainee listens to white noise. Detainee goes to bathroom and is exercised while hooded …

Day 33—December 25, 2002

0230: Interrogator poured one half bottle of water over detainee's head and yelled that the detainee was not in control in the booth, that the interrogator decided everything that happened to him, but the detainee could take the power away by simply telling the truth. Detainee yelled back that the interrogator did this to him and the rest of the bottle was poured over the detainee's head to illustrate the point that the interrogator was in control …

0300: Detainee offered water and refused. Interrogator poured some water on detainee's head … Detainee started falling asleep so interrogator had detainee stand up for 30 minutes … Detainee was subjected to white noise (music) waiting for his IVs to be completed.

Box 2: Selected excerpts from medical ethics codes

United Nations General Assembly—Principles of Medical Ethics Relevant to the Protection of Prisoners Against Torture (1982)[39]

It is a gross contravention of medical ethics, … for health personnel, particularly physicians, to [1] engage, actively or passively, in acts which constitute participation in, complicity in, incitement to or attempts to commit torture or other cruel, inhuman or degrading treatment or punishment, … [2] be involved in any professional relationship with prisoners or detainees the purpose of which is not solely to evaluate, protect or improve their physical and mental health, … [3] (a) apply their knowledge and skills in order to assist in the interrogation of prisoners … in a manner that may adversely affect the physical or mental health or condition of such prisoners …; (b) certify, or to participate in the certification of, the fitness of prisoners … for any form of treatment or punishment that may adversely affect their physical or mental health … or to participate in any way in the infliction of any such treatment or punishment …, [4] participate in any procedure for restraining a prisoner … unless such a procedure is determined in accordance with purely medical criteria as being necessary for the protection of the physical or mental health or the safety of the prisoner or detainee himself … and presents no hazard to his physical or mental health.

World Medical Association—Guidelines for Physicians Concerning Torture and Other Cruel, Inhuman or Degrading Treatment or Punishment in Relation to Detention and Imprisonment [Declaration of Tokyo] (1975)[40]

—The doctor's fundamental role is to alleviate the distress of his or her fellow men, and no motive whether personal, collective or political shall prevail against this higher purpose.

—The doctor shall not countenance, condone or participate in the practice of torture or other forms of cruel, inhuman or degrading procedures, whatever the offence of which the victim of such procedure is suspected, accused or guilty, and whatever the victim's belief or motives, and in all situations, including armed conflict and civil strife.

—The doctor shall not provide any premises, instruments, substances or knowledge to facilitate the practice of torture or other forms of cruel, inhuman or degrading treatment or to diminish the ability of the victim to resist such treatment. The doctor shall not be present during any procedure during which torture or other forms of cruel, inhuman or degrading treatment are used or threatened.

American Psychiatric Association (2006)[41]

No psychiatrist should participate directly in the interrogation of persons held in custody …. Direct participation includes being present in the interrogation room, asking or suggesting questions, or advising authorities on the use of specific techniques of interrogation with particular detainees. However, psychiatrists may provide training to military or civilian investigative or law enforcement personnel on recognizing and responding to persons with mental illnesses, on the possible medical and psychological effects of particular techniques and conditions of interrogation, and on other areas within their professional expertise.

American Medical Association (2006)[42]

Physicians must neither conduct nor directly participate in an interrogation, because a role as physician-interrogator undermines the physicians' role as healer and thereby erodes trust in both the individual physician-interrogator and in the medical profession. Physicians should not monitor interrogations with the intention of intervening in the process, because this constitutes direct participation in interrogation. Physicians may participate in developing effective interrogation strategies that are not coercive but are humane and respect the rights of individuals. When physicians have reason to believe that interrogations are coercive, they must report their observations to the appropriate authorities. If authorities are aware of coercive interrogations but have not intervened, physicians are ethically obligated to report the offenses to independent authorities that have the power to investigate or adjudicate such allegations.

REFERENCES

1. Wittes B, Wyne Z. *The Current Detainee Population of Guantánamo: an empirical study.* Washington, DC: The Brookings Institute; 2008. Available at: www.brookings. edu/~/media/Files/rc/reports/2008/1216_detainees_wittes/1216_detainees_wittes. pdf (accessed October 1, 2009).
2. Physicians for Human Rights. *Break them down: systematic use of psychological torture by U.S. forces.* Cambridge: Physicians for Human Rights; 2005.
3. The Red Cross. *ICRC report on the treatment of 14 "high value detainees" in CIA custody.* Geneva: International Committee of the Red Cross; 2007.
4. www.aclu.org/safefree/index.html
5. Physicians for Human Rights, op. cit.
6. a) Physicians for Human Rights. *Aiding Torture: health professionals' ethics and human rights violations revealed in the May 2004 CIA Inspector General's Report.* 2009.
   b) Huck RA. U.S. Southern Command confidentiality policy for interactions between health care providers and enemy persons under U.S. control, detained in conjunction with Operation Enduring Freedom [memorandum]; August 6, 2002.
   c) Clark PA. Medical Ethics at Guantanamo Bay and Abu Ghraib: the problem of dual loyalty. *Journal of Law, Medicine & Ethics.* 2006; **34**(3): 570–80.
   d) Bloche G, Marks J. Doctors and interrogators at Guantanamo Bay. *NEJM.* 2005; **353**: 6–8.
   e) Bloche G, Marks J. When doctors go to war. *NEJM.* **352**: 1497–99. Miles S. Abu Ghraib: its legacy for military medicine. *The Lancet.* 2004; **364**: 725–9.
7. a) Zagorin A, Duffy M. Inside the interrogation of detainee 063. *TIME.* Jun 12, 2005. Available at: www.time.com/time/magazine/article/0,9171,1071284,00.html (accessed September 1, 2009).
   b) Sands P. *Torture Team: Rumsfeld's memo and the betrayal of American values.* New York, NY: Allen Lane; 2008.
   c) Miles S. Medical ethics and the interrogation of Guantanamo 063. *The American Journal of Bioethics.* 2007: **7**(4): 5.
8. Physicians for Human Rights, The American Red Cross, www.aclu.org, op. cit.
9. Office of Inspector General. *Special Review: counterterrorism detention and interrogation activities (September 2001–October 2003).* May 7, 2004. Available at: www.aclu.org/ oigreport (accessed October 1, 2009).
10. United Nations. *Convention against Torture and Other Cruel, Inhuman and Degrading Treatment or Punishment.* UN; 1984.
11. UN General Assembly. *The Universal Declaration of Human Rights.* UN; 1948.

12. Geneva Convention. *Convention (III), relative to the Treatment of Prisoners of War.* International Committee of the Red Cross; 1949. Available at: www.icrc.org/ihl.nsf/ FULL/375 (accessed April 4, 2011)

13. United Nations General Assembly. *Resolution 45/111.* December 14, 1990.

14. US Army Field Manual. *Interrogation and the Interrogator* [Chapter 1, 34–52]. 1987. Available at: www.globalsecurity.org/intell/library/policy/army/fm/fm34-52 (accessed October 1, 2009).

15. World Medical Association. *Declaration of Tokyo.* WMA; 1975. [*See* Box 2.] Available at: www.wma.net/en/30publications/10policies/c18/index.html (accessed April 4, 2011).

16. Annas GJ. Military medical ethics: Physician first, last, always. *NEJM.* 2008; **359**: 1087–90.

17. a) Physicians for Human Rights. *Dual Loyalty in Health and Professional Practice: proposed guidelines and institutional mechanisms.* Cambridge, Massachusetts; 2002.
    b) Benatar SR, Upshur RE. Dual loyalty of physicians in the military and in civilian life. *Am J Public Health.* 2008; **98**(12): 2161–7.
    c) Howe, EG. Dilemmas in military medical ethics since 9/11. *Kennedy Inst Ethics J.* 2003 Jun; **13**(2): 175–88.

18. The United States Constitution. *Excessive bail shall not be required, nor excessive fines imposed, nor cruel and unusual punishments inflicted* [Article 8].

19. Xenakis SN. Doctors must be healers. *Seton Hall Law Rev.* 2007; **37**(3): 703–10.

20. Howe EG, Kosaraju A, Laraby PR, *et al.* Guantanamo: ethics, interrogation, and forced feeding. *Mil Med.* 2009 Jan; **174**(1): iv–xiii.

21. Public letter to Senator John McCain. October 3, 2005. Available at: www. globalsecurity.org/military/library/news/2005/10/051003-letter-to-sen-mccain.htm (accessed September 1, 2009).

22. a) Lifton R. *The Nazi Doctors: medical killing and the psychology of genocide.* London: Basic Books; 1986.
    b) Nicholl DJ, Jenkins T, Miles SH, *et al.* Biko to Guantanamo: 30 years of medical involvement in torture [letter]. *The Lancet.* 2007; **370**: 823.
    c) Amnesty International. *Under Constant Medical Supervision: torture, ill-treatment and the health professions in Israel and the Occupied Territories.* London: Amnesty International; 1996.
    d) Bamber H, Gordon E, Heilbronn R, *et al.* Attitudes to Torture. *J R Soc Med.* 2002; **95**: 271–2.

23. US Defense Department. *Working group report on detainee interrogations in the global war on terrorism: assessment of legal, historical, policy and operational considerations.* April 4, 2003. Available at: http://en.wikisource.org/wiki/Working_Group_Report_ on_Detainee_Interrogations (accessed October 1, 2009).
    Office of Assistant Attorney General. *Standards of Conduct for Interrogation Under 18 U.S.C. 2340-2340A* [memorandum]. August 1, 2002. Available at: http://www.aclu. org/safefree/torture/25351pub20060427.html (accessed October 1, 2009).

24. Yoo J. Commentary: Behind the "torture memos." *UC Berkeley News.* Jan 4, 2005. Available at: http://berkeley.edu/news/media/releases/2005/01/05_johnyoo.shtml (accessed October 1, 2009).

25. Bush GW. *Memorandum for the Vice President on Humane Treatment of al-Qaeda and Taliban Detainees.* Jun 17, 2004. Available at: http://en.wikisource.org/wiki/

Humane_Treatment_of_al_Qaeda_and_Taliban_Detainees (accessed October 1, 2009).

26. Gonzales AR. *Decision RE: application of the Geneva Conventions to the conflict in Afghanistan* [memorandum]. Jan 25, 2002. In: Greenberg KJ, Dratel JL. *The Torture Papers: the road to Abu Ghraib.* Cambridge: Cambridge University Press; 2005.

27. *Hamdan v. Rumsfeld*, 548 US 557 (2006).

28. Clarkson F. *The Psychologists of Torture.* Psyche, Science and Society [blog]. 2009. Available at: http://psychoanalystsopposewar.org/blog/2009/04/23 (accessed October 1, 2009).

29. Physicians for Human Rights. *Leave No Marks: enhanced interrogation techniques and the risk of criminality.* Available at: http://physiciansforhumanrights.org/library/report-2007-08-02.html (accessed March 17, 2011).

30. Gross ML. *Torture, Ill-Treatment, and Interrogation.* Cambridge, Massachusetts: The MIT Press; 2006. 211–43.

31. American Psychological Association Report. *Presidential Task Force on Psychological Ethics and National Security.* Washington, DC: APA; 2005. Available at: www.apa.org/pubs/info/reports/pens.pdf (accessed April 4, 2011).

32. Silove D. Review of Combating Torture: a manual for action [Amnesty International, London, 2003]. *The Lancet.* 2004; **363**: 1915–16.

33. American Medical Association. *Code of Medical Ethics, Opinion 2.068: physician participation in interrogation.* Chicago, Illinois: American Medical Association; 2006.

34. Rubenstein L. First, Do No Harm. *Seton Hall Law Rev.* 2007; **37**(3): 711–33.

35. Hotez PJ. Reinventing Guantanamo: from detainee facility to center for research on neglected diseases of poverty in the Americas. *PLoS Negl Trop Dis.* 2008. 2(2).

36. Rubenstein LS, Annas GJ. Medical ethics at Guantanamo Bay detention centre and in the US military: a time for reform. *The Lancet.* 2009; **374**: 353–5.

37. Xenakis, op. cit.

38. Sands, op. cit.

39. United Nations. *Principles of Medical Ethics relevant to the Role of Health Personnel, particularly Physicians, in the Protection of Prisoners and Detainees against Torture and Other Cruel, Inhuman, or Degrading Treatment or Punishment.* General Assembly Resolution 37/194. December 18, 1982.

40. World Medical Association, op. cit.

41. American Psychiatric Association. *Principles of Medical Ethics.* Available at: www.psych.org/MainMenu/PsychiatricPractice/Ethics/ResourcesStandards.aspx (accessed October 2, 2009).

42. American Medical Association. *Code of Medical Ethics.* Available at: www.ama-assn.org/ama/no-index/physician-resources/2498.shtml (accessed October 2, 2009).

CHAPTER 10

Risk and shared decision-making: questions of medical practice and social policy in the UK

Sarah A. Lee

THE ISSUES

Risk decision-making in health care is a complex process, requiring careful consideration of burdens and benefits of various options available in any given situation. Medical risk assessment is often institutionally determined and uniformly implemented without regard to individual needs and preferences. If decisions about risk are to be meaningful, the process of balancing the relevant factors needs to acknowledge that individual patient preferences, goals and values vary widely from one person to another. Unfortunately, centralized health care decision-making too often results in blanket responses when dealing with problems to do with risk.

Such top-down decision-making is often driven by perceived needs to meet targets set by government more than any evaluation of likely individual patient outcomes. Policies increasingly work this way, and fear of blame sometimes precipitates knee-jerk reactions that result in risk aversion and general restrictions that can have a direct and potentially negative impact on patient care. Meaningful engagement in issues of risk is often inhibited by the precautionary response of policy-makers, and by physician fear of negative outcomes that reflect poorly on their performance scores. In addition, physicians' fear of litigation may be influenced by perceptions of a heightened litigious medical culture, and risk assessment that is done in a protocol-driven manner can undermine patient-centered care.

BACKGROUND

The British NHS, created in 1948, was the first health system in the West to provide universal, comprehensive, health care provision-free at the point of need. This single-payer system was prefaced on the need to exercise centralized authority. While this is changing, the top-down nature of policy decision-making meant that providers of health care (such as hospitals and primary care centers) made decisions on behalf of the recipients of health care, i.e. patients. This implied an inherently paternalistic system, but with the structure of the NHS now different from the time of its inception, goals for the NHS are moving towards increased decentralization. The the trend towards giving power to local authorities, a recent phenomenon, makes the old "command and control" systems begin to look out of place, especially when viewed against systems operating in other European countries.

Government and regulatory agencies relevant to this discussion include the Department of Health (DH), the National Institute for Clinical Excellence (NICE), the Medicines and Healthcare Products Regulatory Agency (MHRA), and the General Medical Council (GMC). DH is part of central government and is ultimately responsible for running the NHS, while NICE and the MHRA are quasi-independent. The GMC derives its authority from Parliament, yet it is independent of government. While these structures work at national level, decentralization initiatives are in line with the desire to modernise the NHS, reflecting the trend towards patient-centered care and respect for patient autonomy.[1] However, an inherently centralized style of governance still inhibits the introduction of the true individualization of clinical medicine, and against this background this chapter identifies and discusses some of the difficulties around individualizing patient risk and further promoting shared clinical decision-making within the NHS.[2]

SHARED DECISIONS

Shared decision-making ought to lead to a process that incorporates shared evaluation about the management of risk. In spite of its obvious importance, good risk assessment and management is an area of clinical medicine that still tends to be neglected. With the focus of clinical medicine increasingly towards patient-centered care, customized treatment plans ought to be achievable in a way that respects individual patient needs, values and preferences, thereby maximizing patients' ability to make decisions about their health care. While some policymakers recognize the importance of individualized medicine, parallel steps towards individualizing the process of the assessment and management of risk have not yet been taken.

Challenges are encountered at governmental, regulatory, and individual levels, and macro decision-making can find itself in conflict with individualized medical decision-making. Common institutional responses to risk by government policymakers traditionally involve formulaic, top-down approaches, influenced partly by the perceived need to set and meet targets, while limiting negative outcomes.

However, risk-averse, blanket regulation policies preclude the consideration of individual, value-laden factors. Regulatory policy can place pressure on physicians to meet target-driven, performance-based goals in a way that can undermine physician incentives to engage in more individualized approaches to risk. Furthermore, a growing perception of increasing litigation amongst physicians is creating a drive towards defensive medical practices. Subsequent risk aversion can lead to the inhibition if not the prohibition of meaningful discussion about risk.

Simplistic views on assessing risk during the clinical encounter can lead to equating risk assessment and risk management with the mere communication of statistics. What results then is a failure to recognize that both perceptions of risk and the degree of risk acceptability are inherently value-laden, individual and specific. As a result, patients do not always receive critically evaluated scientific evidence that is communicated in a meaningful way to them.

PUBLIC POLICY BARRIERS

The NHS relies on public funds, which means there has to be an element of centralization in terms of accountability.[3] Hence, there is a tendency to try to eliminate risk for fear of condemnation that government is not "providing" the public with adequate safety, and that as a result, the NHS will lose public trust.

NHS regulatory agencies sometimes look to the precautionary principle to handle uncertainty. This can be described as referring to:

> "When an activity raises threats of harm to human health or the environment, precautionary measures should be taken even if some cause and effect relationships are not fully established scientifically. In this context the proponent of an activity, rather than the public, should bear the burden of proof."[4]

Although the precautionary principle is useful and in some cases necessary to protect the public from potentially severe and irreversible harm, it is sometimes applied in situations where clinical uncertainty could be handled through more critical evaluation of data, increased surveillance and follow-up of patients, and vigilant clinical management, all of which need to be on a case-by-case basis. This position is unsatisfactory and unethical if the precautionary principle is used to justify avoiding engaging in the subtle weighing and balancing of unquantifiable variables, which should be integral to the art of shared decision-making about medical risk.

CASE EXAMPLE

The MHRA's handling of the uncertain risks associated with serotonin-specific reuptake inhibitors (SSRIs) in children under the age of 18 provides an example of this risk-averse decision-making. In 2004, the MHRA issued a warning against the use of SSRIs in children and young people,[5] based on reports that SSRIs were associated with increased suicidal behavior, and that for some patients it had minimal effectiveness. Suicidal behavior included increased agitation and arousal, suicidal ideation, and acts of self harm. The MHRA's action created intense controversy, and some child psychiatrists felt that the agency had not adequately studied the data, and instead had imposed generalized restrictions where individual-specific analyses of risks and benefits were really what were needed.

An American paper in the same year questioned the internal and external validity of the evidence,[6] in which psychiatrists from the University of Pittsburgh Medical Center contended that in terms of the available evidence, the quality of research design was poor, the statistical significance was questionable, the data was not stratified in relation to age or severity, there existed no standardized definition of suicidality, and there was inadequate monitoring of adherence to an appropriate treatment regime. Moreover, the relative risk of non-treatment was not addressed within the comparative research trials.[7] As Jonathan Green, child and adolescent psychiatrist at the University of Manchester, states, *"The possibility that good-quality medical management and surveillance could obviate any putative risk was not included in the balance."*[8] The MHRA's handling of the SSRI issue ignited the debate on why regulatory agencies handle clinical uncertainty with reflexive prohibition instead of addressing the underlying issues. This approach needs to be replaced by carefully implementing customized treatment plans, complete with vigilant follow-up and new, unbiased, rigorously designed research.

NEGATIVE OUTCOMES AND TARGET-DRIVEN POLICY

In a 2005 lecture, Nuffield Trust Professor Mike Pringle spoke of *"two ideologies fighting for the soul of British medicine."* At issue, he said, is:

> "Whether the new culture of health care will be to regain but essentially maintain our long tradition of medical paternalism; or whether it will be to maximise patient care and choice, to protect patients from harm and to promote a patient-centred, patient-led healthcare system."[9]

In order to improve public perception that government is fulfilling its role of "guaranteeing" safety, regulatory and government agencies increasingly tend to focus on achieving statistical targets based on minimizing negative outcomes rather than on maximizing positive outcomes. Statistics can be reported to the public by the media but the problem is that government tends not to trust individuals to make good choices, which can lead to policymakers becoming preoccupied with auditing performance instead of critically examining a system's effectiveness.

The problems are these: Firstly, target-based risk management largely involves unidirectional communication, and it lacks patient views and feedback. Secondly, target-based regulation is often at the expense of long-term gains that can be attained when freedom, choice and customized treatment are the main focus. This would make targets difficult to measure, and it is possible for policy aimed at minimizing negative outcomes to lose sight of unreported and perhaps less tangible or less easily measured positive outcomes and gains that can be achieved when risk evaluation is more individual. While this policy, when applied to orthopedic surgery, for example, may decrease the number of falls and optimize patients' postoperative recovery by not sending them home too soon, it does not take account of increased incidences of depression and dementia that arise when patients are removed from their social support and familiar surroundings for extended periods of time.

This approach does not allow individual patients and care providers to assess whether the risks of living at home might outweigh the benefits—an assessment that should be based on a patient's mental status and capacity, the availability of resources (including social support), and the needs, preferences and values of the individual patient. The Department of Health guidance titled *Independence, Choice and Risk: a guide to best practice in supported decision making* (2007) talks about the importance of *"person-centred treatment plans"* and taking a *"positive approach to risk."*[10] But in order for these recommendations to be realized, there needs to be more room for debate on how policymakers and regulators can better allow for individualized risk assessment and management.

OBSTACLES TO INDIVIDUALIZING CLINICAL RISK

The culture of performance assessment through target setting extends down to the level of the individual physician, and it can have a real effect on the clinical encounter. For example, surgeons have been under pressure to report individual performance scores, resulting in a drive towards more risk-averse practice. Surgeon performance scores are determined by assessing a patient's postoperative outcome in relation to a patient's previously calculated risk score (calculated by determining a numerical value for each risk factor, e.g. age, sex, medical comorbidities, etc.—the cumulative value of the individual risk factors represents a patient's overall risk of mortality). The problem lies in the fact that risk scores have increased significantly over the past decade (a primary factor being the demographics of an aging population), together with the fact that in high-risk patients the risk score can *under* estimate a patient's actual risk.

For example, in a case where a patient is about to undergo a carotid endarterectomy (CEA), a procedure to remove the inner lining of a partially blocked carotid artery to increase blood flow, the surgeon's evaluation of a patient's medical profile must be individual-specific. A patient's actual risk can be misrepresented because when a patient has already undergone triple bypass surgery, this greatly increases the risk of complications due to a previous history of disease. This needs to be captured in order to obtain an accurate picture of risk for this category of patient. Risk points that do not allocate scores for previous disease complications put this type of patient at high risk of postoperative complication and death because of a misleading profile of risk. Risk points need to be added to the patient's score to account for the underlying disease separately from the risks associated with the CEA. If a patient were to undergo back-to-back procedures, it is perfectly possible for this additional risk to be overlooked, giving an unduly optimistic risk score for the procedure taken on its own.

When trying to formularize patient risk, actual risk can be underestimated to the extent that can influence a surgeon's willingness to undertake the procedure, e.g. by trying to maintain high performance score figures. Another factor to take into account is a cardiac surgeon's experience in terms of the numbers of times that s/he has performed the procedure. Overall, it is not in either the surgeon's nor the patient's best interests to ignore an elevated compound risk.

LITIGIOUS CULTURES AND DEFENSIVE PRACTICE

Another factor that can influence clinical risk decision-making is the fear of litigation on the part of the physician. Perceptions of an escalating litigious medical culture can exert an additional pressure, pointing towards risk-averse, defensive medical practice. Although there has not been a significant increase in the number of litigation cases over recent years, around 10% of the NHS' total budget is currently spent by the National Health Service Litigation Authority (NHSLA). Moreover, there has been almost a nine-fold increase in the amount of money paid out during settlements (both in and out of the courts) over the past nine years.[11]

One can argue that fear of heightened litigation in the UK has been, in part, a reaction to the way in which the courts have handled cases involving failure to warn. In the past, physicians were partly protected from prosecution for failure to warn of a particular materialized risk if a defendant could prove that the patient's decision would not have been different even if the patient had been informed of the risk prior to treatment (proof of causation). Since the landmark case of Chester v. Afshar in 2004, there has been a raised burden of expectation on physicians to warn against remote, unlikely but material risks. This case was significant in that the adjudication suggests that proof of causation is no longer necessary in order for a physician to be found negligent for failing to warn about such risk.[12]

This level of disclosure is reflected in current General Medical Council (UK) guidelines, which state that:

"[The physician] must tell patients if an investigation or treatment might result in a serious adverse outcome, even if the likelihood is very small. [The physician] should also tell patients about less serious side effects or complications if they occur frequently, and explain what the patient should do if they experience any of them."[13]

Some fear that increased burdens on physicians to warn against a potentially indefinite number of risks when seeking to obtain consent will lead towards defensive practices and risk-aversive decision-making when dealing with high-risk treatments and procedures. However, there is no clear evidence to support this.

RISK COMMUNICATION

Poor risk communication poses a potential barrier to patient-centered risk management, and there is a lingering perception that the "expert" is somehow privileged to the knowledge, and that lay persons cannot properly understand and assimilate information needed in order to reach a decision. Such perceptions can lead to a lack of emphasis on meaningful dialogue or openness in communications between physicians and patients. Patients can therefore be left under-informed, feeling disempowered in the decision-making process, with the possible consequence that patients seek information from other sources that may not be accurate or reliable.

In 2001 the Department of Health in London commissioned a study *"to identify and understand individuals' risk literacy and its impact upon risk information requirements."*[14] The largest case study was based on public reaction to the controversy over the measles/mumps/rubella (MMR) vaccination, which had been rumored to cause inflammatory bowel syndrome and autism in children. A degree of public frenzy then resulted in fewer children than anticipated being vaccinated. While there was heated concern over the MMR vaccine, only 40% of participants in the study had seen any Department of Health-issued information on the vaccine (in spite of having ready access to the Internet). Parents expressed surprise and anger that they had not been informed about literature that was directly relevant to their children's health and exposure to risk. They also felt a lack of control when it came to accessing official government sanctioned information. Despite feeling trust towards physicians, parents said they often hesitated to ask questions or request further information, in part because they did not feel their family doctor had time to discuss these things. Many parents received their information from stories through the media, and overall, parents expressed confusion and difficulty rationalizing and trying to reach a decision.

The Department of Health study determined that the issue of choice was a predominant concern among parents. Regardless of whether they had chosen for or against vaccination, many parents reported that they felt they ought to have been given more choice and more information in order to support their decisions. Because parents felt they were being denied the opportunity to choose, they viewed their relationship with government authority as more antagonistic than collaborative. The lack of readily accessible, reliable information resulted in the suspicion that government was either concealing a conspiracy, or that the MMR vaccine was part of a scheme to increase cost-effectiveness rather than the intended goal of increased compliance. Public perceptions of risk may not always be well founded, in terms of rationality and being evidence based, but they ought not to be ignored. It may be better to trust the public than to try and control information in a way that leaves room for doubts and suspicions to grow, even if the science itself is not completely devoid of ambiguity.

IMPLICATIONS FOR FUTURE NHS POLICY

Policymakers ought to rely less on restrictive blanket policies and instead leave room for case-by-case assessment based on individual factors. Optimizing patient safety need not mean inhibiting individual decision-making. At a 2006 lecture, the National Director for Patients and the Public at the Department of Health stated that:

> "Regulation should exist not to protect us from uncertainty, but to enable us to make choices with understanding. Not to stop companies, researchers, doctors, and patients from taking risks but to enable risks to be taken for individual and public good. Regulation saves lives; but lives lived are enabled by risk."[15]

Safety measures should be focused on attaining more critically evaluated and comprehensive research data that allow clinicians to better risk-stratify their patients and balance potential burdens and benefits of treatment against non-treatment. Safety measures need to involve careful clinical management and vigilant follow-up to guard against signs of harm and to monitor treatment effectiveness. Policymakers and governance bodies should not rely on general, numerical, one-dimensional targets as the sole indicator of effectiveness. Evaluation of patient care must include a multidimensional assessment of whether a proposed treatment plan addresses a patient's values, needs and preferences; this should be considered a routine part of patient-centered care.

Individualization of risk assessment requires a greater focus on patient-centered regulation, which means creating opportunities for engagement of public and patients in making risk-associated decisions. In order to remove the expert/non-expert barrier, health policymakers ought to ensure that accessible, easily identifiable, understandable information is made available to the public. Furthermore, the dissemination of information needs to be done in a timely manner before the public looks to other less-reliable sources. Providing access to information in a meaningful and contextualized manner should help to foster trust between regulators and the public, empowering individuals by granting them a sense of responsibility by being more in control of their own health issues.

Moreover, engaging the public requires not just that information flows from policymakers to the public, but that there is a proper two-way dialogue. The public needs to have an avenue of communication through which they can voice concerns, ask questions and give feedback during the different phases of policy development. People with different backgrounds and levels of understanding of science and risk need to have access to and be able to assimilate information in a meaningful way. By consulting a diverse number of people, policymakers can identify confusion and clarify any inaccurate perceptions that are prevalent among the public (such as questions regarding causational links between MMR and autism).

Some of these arguments apply to public policy on vaccination programs for "swine flu," or the H1N1 virus. While there have been few concerns about safety, and quantities of information have made available to the general public, at the time of writing it is not certain that the public is any better equipped to decide whether or not to go ahead and have the vaccination. Lack of confidence in government data and uncertainty about perceptions of risk would seem to be key factors.

Sir David Weatherall, Chancellor of Keele University and renowned microbiologist, argued in a spoken address (2009) that the future of medicine is *"trending towards individualizing medical therapy through the exploration of genomics"*, saying that progress made in the individualization of the science of medicine needs to be paralleled by the individualization of the art of medicine. Whether this goal is likely to be achieved depends partly on the extent to which clinical policymakers, regulators and the public trust government and can come to a better understanding about how to contextualize risk.

REFERENCES

1. Goodrich J, Cornwall J. *Seeing the person in the patient: the Point of Care review paper.* London: The King's Fund Report; 2008.
2. Klein R. *The New Politics of the NHS.* Oxford: Radcliffe Publishing Ltd; 2006.
3. Ibid.
4. Ashford N, Barrett K, Bernstein A, *et al. Wingspread Statement on the Precautionary Principle.* Kobe Global Development Research Center; 1998.
5. Report of the Committee on Safety of Medicines Working Group on the Safety of *Selective Serotonin Reuptake Inhibitors* London, England; 2004. Available at: www.mhra.gov.uk/home/groups/pl-p/documents/drugsafetymessage/con019472.pdf (accessed April 4, 2011).
6. Brent DA, Birmaher B. British warnings on SSRIs questioned. *J Am Acad Child Adolesc Psychiatry.* 2004; **43**(4): 379–80.
7. Ibid.
8. Green J. Avoiding a spiral of precaution in mental healthcare. *Advances in Psychiatric Treatment.* 2006; **12**: 1–4.
9. Pringle M. Revalidation of doctors: the credibility challenge. *The John Fry Fellowship Lecture.* London: The Nuffield Trust; 2005.
10. Department of Health. *Independence, Choice and Risk: a guide to best practice in supported decision making.* Available at: www.dh.gov.uk/en/Publicationsandstatistics/Publications/PublicationsPolicyAndGuidance/DH_076511 (accessed September 14, 2009).

11. NHS Litigation Factsheet No. 2. 2008. Available at: www.nhsla.com/NR/rdonlyres/465D7ABD-239F-4273-A01E-C0CED557453D/0/NHSLAFactsheet2financial information200708.doc (accessed September 14, 2009).

12. Chester v. Afshar. 2004 UKHL 41. Available at: www.bailii.org/uk/cases/UKHL/2004/41.html (accessed September 14, 2009).

13. General Medical Council (UK). *Consent: patients and doctors making decisions together*. 2008. Available at: www.gmc-uk.org/guidance/ethical_guidance/consent_guidance/Consent_guidance.pdf (accessed April 4, 2011).

14. Petts J, Wheeley S, Homan J, *et al. Risk Literacy and the Public—MMR, Air Pollution and Mobile Phones* [report for the Department of Health]. January 2003. Birmingham, UK: University of Birmingham.

15. Cayton H. *All for the Best? Risk, Regulation and Choice in Healthcare* [the second MHRA annual lecture]. London; 2006.

CHAPTER 11

Italian policy and the ethics of ECT

Anthony Marfeo

INTRODUCTION

In April 1938, Ugo Cerletti performed the world's first electroconvulsive treatment (ECT) for a patient with catatonia, and it brought good results.[1] However, nearly 60 years later a national ethics body in Italy was charged with deciding whether "as a precautionary measure" the practice of ECT should be suspended.[2] Over time the pendulum swung in different directions, and recently there have been signs that ECT may again have to be evaluated. These changing views have resulted from public perceptions of ECT as much as from clinical and scientific data.

ECT is often referred to in the literature as being the most effective treatment for bringing about remission in cases of depression, particularly in severe cases. Why then do many developed nations use it sparingly, and with more controversy than almost any other treatment? Legal frameworks for providing this type of care display regional, national and international variation, and public opinion polls show varying results. Worldwide, the public seems to have only limited understanding about this form of treatment and its potential uses, and the entertainment media fill the gap with sensationalistic portrayals of ECT. These usually feature idiosyncratic characters who display behavioral characteristics that are at odds with the bio-psychosocial models of mental health disease that are presently dominant in Western medical culture.

CLINICAL DATA OVERVIEW

Detailed discussion of the clinical scenarios in which ECT might be used is beyond the scope of this paper; however, use of ECT has been attempted for many psychiatric illnesses over a period spanning seven decades. The most reliable data shows that it works quite well with depressive-spectrum disorders, including depression with psychotic features, as well as with catatonia.[3] The cost-effectiveness of ECT versus more pharmacotherapeutic interventions has not been shown to be significantly different, but the evidence is not yet conclusive, making policy decision-making on this issue especially challenging. Of note is the fact that a full course of ECT can be accomplished more quickly when compared with the amount of time required to achieve a response to treatment using medications.

One reason ECT is not used more frequently is that the side effects of treatment can be problematic. Memory loss, particularly for events during the episode of illness and treatment with ECT, is the most commonly reported and distressing adverse event. Modern alterations in technique have been primarily aimed at decreasing the incidence and severity of this amnesia. In the early years of ECT use, induced seizures sometimes caused bone fractures and painful muscle contractions, but widespread use of anesthetics has dramatically reduced the incidence of adverse musculoskeletal reaction. Some patients, such as the medically frail, the elderly, and some pregnant women, could actually face fewer side effects with ECT than with a pharmacological form of therapy.

For most people, ECT carries a higher risk of serious side effects than many, though not all, pharmacological therapies. However, the risks are immaterial if viewed out of context, and this is why it is worth considering the benefits as well as the risks and burdens of treatment in particular settings, having in mind that for some patients, the benefits could be substantially more than with any other single therapy approach. Diseases that are being treated with ECT are potentially life-threatening and might not be self-limited, which leads to interesting and challenging issues about when to use these high-risk but high-reward treatments.

Each nation, state and professional body approaches this question in a slightly different manner, consistent with relevant local policy and legal frameworks. Complicating the matter further are questions relating to public opinion and politics, which are often based on unreliable sources of information, further colored by a range of personal, social and moral frameworks. In order to explore these frameworks in context, the Italian health care system will be discussed briefly, in order to try and establish the logic and reasoning behind this type of treatment decision.

ITALIAN *SERVIZIO SANITARIO NAZIONALE* (SSN)

The Italian SSN was established in 1978, and it was modeled closely on the British NHS.[5] According to the Italian Constitution, the Italian state is responsible for health care provision, although recent reforms have mostly delegated control of health care issues to the 20 regional health authorities. These authorities are funded primarily by national taxes and supplemented with local taxes. Essentially, the state sets the minimum levels of care that are to be provided. The regions are responsible for structuring the management and provision of care, and they enjoy a high degree of autonomy. ECT is not specifically listed as a required benefit, but the care of patients with mental health problems is included in SSN catalogues listing benefits that should be equally available in all the regions.[6]

Considerable North-South disparities exist, due to economic differences between the wealthier Northern and poorer Southern states. Northern regions contribute twice the amount of region-specific tax funds, and regional infrastructures tend to have difficulties in pulling out of this cycle. This is partly due to "health tourism" that goes from South to North, and which is compensated for by retroactive payments between the regions.[7] Health care funding is supplied at the national level, but clinical decisions and responsibilities are largely decentralized. In response to this, the *Istituto Superiore di Sanita* was created as a central, national body, one of its responsibilities being to ensure that devices and treatments meet safety standards.[8] A second institute, the *Consiglio Superiore di Sanita*, was established to form ad hoc groups of consultants who could make evidence-based recommendations.[9] There are many such consulting groups, representing most of the more controversial or rapidly evolving fields in medicine.[10] Together, these organizations are roughly analogous to the British National Institute for Health and Clinical Excellence (NICE),

COMPARISONS: THE UK AND ITALY

NICE was established in 1999 with the principal aim of encouraging standardization of best practice throughout England and Wales. It reviews both clinical and cost-effectiveness, alongside considerations such as risk. NICE published guidance on ECT in 2003 and took the view that in limited situations ECT was an acceptable treatment. NICE also recognized that within this framework, patient wishes took precedence over clinical recommendations.[11]

Judgment on the effectiveness of ECT was primarily based on a meta-analysis of 119 randomised-controlled trials, and the conclusions reached were broad. ECT was found to work for depression and some types of schizophrenia (particularly catatonic), but overall, ECT should be reserved for severe cases of depression, mania and catatonia, or for use in cases where other treatment options had already failed in treating those conditions. The approach adopted by NICE acknowledges that some groups of people experience more benefit than risks or burdens,[12] and NICE recommended that further research was needed in order to be to help define who these subgroups were.

The NICE recommendations were controversial and were perceived to limit individual patient options. As noted in a subsequent critical editorial, there were no psychiatrists on the advisory board responsible for compiling these recommendations, although the board did consult with psychiatric groups. In addition, finer details such as bilateral versus unilateral electrodes and differences in electricity characteristics were apparently ignored by NICE, and these variations are known to affect the incidence and severity of adverse reactions.[13]

Methodological concerns such as these threaten to undermine the process whereby NICE makes authoritative recommendations on best practice. In 2005 the Royal College of Psychiatrists (RCP) in London published its own ECT handbook for clinicians, and it suggested using ECT as a third-line treatment for cases of refractory depression in addition to indications outlined by NICE. It stated that the use of ECT could be justified in more situations than those explicitly outlined by NICE, thus leaving room for the exercise of clinical judgment.

The handbook goes on to remind clinicians that: *"The NICE guidance on ECT does not have any legal jurisdiction over clinical practice, and its legal significance could be established only if it were cited in a court case."* This was a direct challenge, and as readers will have noted in Chapter 3, the organization was subject to a major reorganization around this time, including reappraisal of the legal validity of its guidance.[14] From an ethical perspective, objectivity is probably key, and it is not clear which set of guidelines is freer of self-interest or outside interference, or more in line with the scientific evidence. In Italy there have been similar legal and political entanglements that have led to a degree of hesitance, explicitly in allowing ECT to be used, and this had a practical effect of denying patients' choice.

BASAGLIA LAW

Italian mental health reforms occurred around the same time as the formation of the SSN in the late 1970s. *Law 180*, passed in 1978, provided for the shift of inpatients from state-run psychiatric hospitals to community-based outpatient centers, and these new centers were to be run by the SSN.[15] Compulsory inpatient treatment was still occasionally allowed, but only for periods of up to seven days. These brief periods were to be sanctioned with approval from two doctors, an elected official and a magistrate; involuntary admissions are still decreasing today and are among the lowest in Europe.[16]

"The Italian Experiment," as it became known internationally, was undertaken in a shifting social atmosphere. In philosophical and scientific terms, an ideological framework emphasizing the importance of environmental and psychosocial factors was gradually displacing belief in biological bases of behavior.[17] A psychiatrist named Franco Basaglia championed these shifts in law and public opinion, and his opinions were widely reflected in the policy and ethical discourse of the time regarding ECT.

ITALIAN ETHICAL DISCOURSE

The Italian head of government formed a National Bioethics Committee (NBC) in March 1990 to represent Italian judicial and ethical thinkers and provide a tool for bioethical decision-making. This corresponds with European and global initiatives supported by the United Nations to establish a national committee for bioethics, with responsibility for monitoring and evaluating ethical aspects of research.[18] The Italian committee's stated goal is to promote:

> "An international-level comparison on the state of the art of biomedical research and genetic engineering which might serve as a valid point of reference for future choices in which the progress of science can be reconciled with the respect for human freedom and dignity."[19]

This NBC consists of 40 interdisciplinary members, who serve for three years each; its published guidelines are not legally binding but provide reliable advice for policymakers, especially at local levels. There are also regional ethics committees, as well as committees in specific hospitals, which are consulted when a patient is under consideration for ECT.[20]

In September of 1995, ECT was investigated by the Commission, which recognized the clinical and evidence-based utility of this treatment. However, they took issue with the difficulty of ensuring the *"safeguarding of a patient's personality and dignity,"*[21] and psychiatrists were vulnerable to being seen as using ECT to *"provide a quick fix ... rather than working together with the patient to understand the sense and nature of that suffering, and thereby provide succour to the patient as a person."*[22]

The Commission also took a biological view into account, accepting the validity of using ECT in certain cases. These include: severe endogenous depression; delirious depression; some severe mania; catatonia; depression with high suicide risk; progressive amentia; any time that medical issues preclude pharmacological management; and, more broadly, whenever a patient is suffering severely. Ultimately, they recommended that ECT could be used on a case-by-case basis with supervision, and in consultation with local ethics committees.[23]

PUBLIC OPINION

It is necessary and reasonable to ask what is causing this discrepancy between clinical data and actual policies and practices, and surveys of attitudes have shown mixed results. Patients who have undergone ECT generally have positive attitudes, as do most psychiatrists regarding the treatment. But psychologists and lay people with less exposure to mental illness tend to have more unfavorable views of ECT.[24] Prior work has shown that media such as film, television and the Internet are a key source of public perceptions regarding some psychiatric therapies. A recent study surveyed 379 people, asking them questions in regard to factual knowledge about ECT, as well as sources of knowledge and attitudes in response to clinical scenarios. Only 57% correctly identified the head as being the stimulation site. More troublesome still is that only 10% of patients were aware that ECT is only performed on anesthetized and unconscious patients. Overall, attitudes toward ECT were unfavorable, with examples of reasons given including "uncomfortable having electric current passed through the head," and ECT as being "too invasive."[25]

Movies such as *One Flew Over the Cuckoo's Nest* were cited as a factor in other national studies; one study noted a decline of 45% in the use of ECT in the USA in the five-year period beginning in 1975, which was the year the film was released.[26] It is tempting to attribute this to influence of the mass media, although it is perhaps more likely that social currents of the time affected medical professionals and patients as well as filmmakers. Future rigorous public opinion surveys may be able to shed more light on this issue. A sample patient vignette will help illustrate usage of the Italian health care system and issues surrounding ECT.

CASE EXAMPLE AND POLICY ANALYSIS

A 40-year-old woman presents to the emergency department psychiatrist with a three-week history of depressed mood, accompanied by insomnia, anorexia and feelings of diffuse guilt. She feels that she has been a failure in life, despite recently completing a graduate degree while teaching full time. She never sought treatment for similar episodes and now feels so hopeless that she is actively considering suicide. Her psychiatrist considers her treatment options, noting the need for rapid improvement and that it would be imprudent to send her home in her current state. Would ECT be useful in this case, and more importantly, would it be possible to provide, given local health care resources and policy frameworks that have been described?

What should our patient expect by way of treatment? In the short term, her psychiatrist is free to guide her towards ECT, and she would be likely to have a quick and positive response. However, there would be a need to consult with a local hospital ethics committee first. Since a pharmaceutical intervention would be a less-involved process, medication could be chosen as the first-line treatment. This patient, having no prior personal exposure to ECT, probably has her own prejudices against this form of treatment, which could influence her ultimate treatment options and decision. Should she be deemed a risk to herself and yet be unwilling to remain under her doctor's care, she could be involuntarily hospitalized. However, this would not be a decision for her doctor alone and would have to include legal opinion and a second clinical evaluation.

Whatever her treatment plan, it would be paid for by the SSN using funds from national and regional taxation, and the burden of her illness would as a result be distributed amongst the other members of her community as well as society as a whole. While the provision of her care is mandated by national government, it is managed by regional government, and depending on the wealth of her particular region, there may be more or less available resources to commit to her care, even though national minimum standards have to be met.

Two questions of policy arise. Firstly, the patient contributes taxes regardless of which services are used, and political pressure to reduce the use of services is unlikely to be experienced directly by the patient. Secondly, regions contribute only a portion of the funds for the services that they choose to provide, and there is an element of federal subsidy, which has the potential to encourage increased provision of services by regional management. Wide regional variations in wealth cause differences in the levels of care that are available, and if she came from a rich northern state, she would have more nearby physicians and hospitals from which to choose than if she came from the South. Furthermore, in the North she may well be offered care that is more costly to provide because of different expectations, despite efforts to standardize care nationally.

Ultimately, our patient ought to receive adequate care for her depression. She will probably recover fully from her episode of depression but she is likely to relapse, as many people do. Her ability to pay will not be a factor in the type of care she receives; however, she would be less likely to receive a particular type of treatment, specifically ECT, depending on where she lives. This is not to say that she would receive the "wrong" treatment, rather that ethical, social, political, policy and financial frameworks could influence her treatment options. In this case, in spite of external constraints and policy considerations, the ultimate outcome is very likely to be acceptable to this patient.

So in this vignette at least, there is a "happy ending," with the patient receiving the care she needs, even if in the first instance, it was not clear whether or not that would include ECT. In summary, it is fair to conclude that policy confusion is not usually in patients' best interests, and that shifting opinions about the use of ECT could potentially result in patients being denied a form of care that for them could be the most effective. Treatment provision in Italy, and possibly in the UK, would depend on resources being available when needed, where patients live, and where the pendulum is pointing at the time.

REFERENCES

1. Passione R. Italian psychiatry in an international context: Ugo Cerletti and the case of electroshock. *Hist Psychiatry.* 2004; **15**(57 Pt 1): 83–104.
2. Italian National Commission on Bioethics. The ethics of electro-shock therapy. *Bull Med Ethics.* May 1996; **118**: 20–2.
3. Abrams R. *Electroconvulsive Therapy.* 4th ed. Oxford and New York: Oxford University Press; 2002.
4. Prudic J, Haskett RF, Mulsant B, *et al.* Resistance to antidepressant medications and short-term clinical response to ECT. *Am J Psychiatry.* Aug 1996; **153**(8): 985–92.
5. France G, Taroni F. The Evolution of Health Policy-making in Italy. *J Health Polit Policy Law.* Feb-Apr 2005; **30**(1–2): 169–87.
6. France G, Taroni F, Donatini A. The Italian Healthcare System. *Health Econ.* Sep 2005; **14**(Suppl 1): 187–202.

7. Ibid.

8. Istituto Superiore di Sanita. Available at: www.iss.it/chis/?lang=2 (accessed September 20, 2009).

9. France G. Health technology assessment in Italy. *Int J Technol Assess Health Care.* 2000; **16**(2): 459–74.

10. Ministero del Lavoro, della Salute e delle Politiche Sociali. Consiglio superiore di sanità. Available at: www.ministerosalute.it/ministero/sezMinistero.jsp?label=css (accessed September 20, 2009).

11. National Institute for Clinical Excellence. *Guidance on the Use of Electroconvulsive Therapy.* London: National Institute for Clinical Excellence; 2003. Available at: www.nice.org.uk/nicemedia/pdf/59ectfullguidance.pdf (accessed September 20, 2009).

13. Cole C, Tobiansky R. Electroconvulsive therapy: NICE guidance may deny many patients treatment that they might benefit from. *BMJ.* 2003; **327**(7415): 621.

14. Royal College of Psychiatrists' Special Committee on ECT. *The ECT Handbook: The third report of the Royal College of Psychiatrists' Special Committee of ECT.* London: Royal College of Psychiatrists; 2005.

15. Morosini P, Veltro F. A critical appraisal of papers describing Italian psychiatric services. *Int J Soc Psychiatry.* Spring 1989; **35**(1): 110–19.

16. Priebe S, Badesconyi A, Fioritti A, *et al.* Re-institutionalisation in mental health care: comparison of data on service provision from six European countries. *BMJ.* 2005; **330**(7483): 123–6.

17. Benaim S. The Italian Experiment. *Psychiatr Bull.* 1983; **17**(1): 7–10.

18. UNESCO. Bioethics. Available at: http://portal.unesco.org/shs/en/ev.php-URL_ID=1372&URL_DO=DO_TOPIC&URL_SECTION=201.html (accessed September 20, 2009).

19. Governo Italiano. *Italian National Bioethics Committee.* Available at: www.governo.it/bioetica/eng (accessed September 20, 2009).

20. Cattorini P, Mordacci R. Ethics committees in Italy. *HEC Forum.* 1992; **4**(3): 219–26.

21. Italian National Commission on Bioethics, op. cit.

22. Ibid.

23. Ibid.

24. Kalayam B, Steinhart MJ. A survey of attitudes on the use of electroconvulsive therapy. *Hosp Community Psychiatr.* Mar 1981; **32**(3): 185–8.

25. Teh SP, Helmes E, Drake DG. A Western Australian survey on public attitudes toward and knowledge of electroconvulsive therapy. *Int J Soc Psychiatr.* May 2007; **53**(3): 247–73.

26. Thompson JW, Weiner RD, Myers CP. Use of ECT in the United States in 1975, 1980, and 1986. *Am J Psychiatr.* Nov 1994; **151**(11): 1657–61.

PART 3

CHAPTER 12

Comparative analysis and future health care decision-making

Our thesis in this book has been that while health policy analysis is often determined by economic and political considerations, ethical dimensions to policy must also be considered. As a corollary to this, failure to consider ethical dimensions in health policy when analyzing the implications for patients regarding changes in health policy and law can lead to policies with inadvertent outcomes, policies that are difficult to enforce, or policies that fail to meet their primary objectives. In order to familiarize readers with this rationale and give an account of philosophical underpinnings and alternative ways of doing policy analysis, Part 1 examined relationships between law, policy and ethics and different frameworks that can be used in policy analysis, with case examples drawn mainly from the UK. Part 2 went on to provide health policy case examples from around the world to illustrate these interactions, taking examples from both developing and developed countries. We also considered concepts extending beyond national borders, such as relationships between medicine and the pharmaceutical industry, public perceptions of risk, and how medical professionalism is affected by external, political considerations.

In Part 3 we begin by comparing and contrasting how health policy, law and ethics interact in these different settings. This will help address the following broad topics that emerged from the case studies in Part II:

1 Changing health care systems
2 Professional standards in a cross-cultural context
3 The legal and regulatory environment
4 Conflicts of interest
5 Integrating public opinion into risk assessment strategies

After addressing these topics, we consider the limitations we encountered in analyzing health policy, law and professional standards in international settings, asking what ethical challenges may be inherent to accomplishing the task of undertaking ethical policy analyses.

CHANGING HEALTH CARE SYSTEMS

A striking element in the chapters on China and Malaysia is the significant changes that are underway regarding the methods by which health care is now financed. In China, the 1978 economic reforms began a process of transforming economic structures from a socialist-planned economy to a more market-based economy. This change involved the health care system, which was transformed from a system of highly subsidized universal access with uneven quality to a mix of part government-supported health care institutions and part fee-for-service type arrangements. Similar though perhaps slower and less extensive change is taking place in Malaysia, where the government is also attempting to move more components of health care away from the public sector. In both countries this change has had significant impacts in terms of access, quality and cost.

i) Access to care

In China, the socialized system of care provided a system of universal access organized around social structures like villages, townships and counties in the rural areas, and neighborhoods in the more urban areas. More recently, fees for access to primary care and most outpatient care remain quite low, and so those services remain quite accessible. Fees for hospital-based services, however, have escalated considerably, with the availability of most hospital-based care being contingent on paying before even entering the hospital. As urban dwellers have more success in gaining higher wages, hospital fees are more difficult for the rural poor to pay. The result is that many rural hospitals have low censuses and therefore low profits from which to improve salaries or purchase new equipment. In contrast, urban hospital systems typically have flourishing state-of-the-art equipment and highly trained physicians. A similar though perhaps less dire situation is present in Malaysia, with urban dwellers with high incomes having access to a wide range of private sector services, and the rural poor finding much difficulty accessing public sector care.

This maldistribution of access to health care, with urban dwellers having better access than those living in rural areas, is a pattern that can be seen in other countries, including countries like the US and India. Clearly, this ethical analysis means that health policies will need to be developed further in order to try and improve health care for the rural poor. The Chinese Health Reform Acts of 2009 provide increased subsidies and insurance products for the rural poor, and Malaysian government efforts to subsidize health care in rural areas are further examples of policies aimed at addressing this inequity.

ii) Quality of care

The differences in quality of care in rural settings and urban settings can be predicted based on the economic differences outlined above. In China, village-level care may be provided by doctors who are largely untrained in Western-style, allopathic medicine. Township and county-level hospitals are often staffed with doctors who have only two or three years of training after high school. Because of economic difficulties, equipment and physical plant conditions in rural hospitals are often sub-optimal. In urban settings, patients are more often cared for by graduates of five-year medical school programs. Urban hospitals, on the other hand, have been quite profitable, and so large building campaigns and purchases of advanced equipment are becoming more common. The quality of care provided in these urban inpatient settings is equivalent to many Western settings, and the situation described here has several similarities to the quality of care that exists in India.

Clearly, equity in access to quality health care between urban and rural populations is an important ethical issue. In both China and Malaysia there are health policies that attempt to address the differences in quality of care. Both countries are trying mandatory rotation of newly trained physicians to work for periods of time in the more remote rural settings. However, physicians are rarely pleased with having to shoulder this duty, and the impact of this policy could be less than anticipated. China is also developing policies to bring rural physicians to urban areas for more hands-on training. This type of program holds promise to improve the quality of care for people living in rural areas, especially where physicians do indeed return to rural areas to practice.

The quality of care in outpatient settings in China affords an opportunity for another interesting ethical discussion. Marienfeld documents patients being seen for only a few minutes during an initial visit in a psychiatric outpatient setting. The abbreviated length of these appointments will have an effect on the quality of the history and physical exam that can be completed. Few follow-up appointments are ever scheduled, and so changes in health status are difficult to achieve and thereby impossible to measure.

Because access to care is so important, fees for outpatient care are kept quite low, meaning that physicians prefer to practice in the more lucrative inpatient settings. The result is that many patients are being seen by few physicians, making the time each patient spends with a physician short and precious. With what might be regarded as suboptimal care being provided, one has to ask if this is unethical; but it is hard to make that argument from an equity standpoint as no one group is being disadvantaged relative to another. Current Chinese health policy appears to value access over quality in the outpatient setting, and changing the reimbursement system to favor outpatient care may help to improve quality in the outpatient setting, but that could come at the expense of access unless government subsidizes the change. These tensions are inbuilt, and so there are no easy fixes.

iii) Cost of care

As noted, the cost of outpatient care remains quite affordable for most Chinese patients and for most Malaysian patients cared for in the public sector. However, in China, the cost of hospitalization for the rural poor is staggering in comparison with their income, which means that even where families pool many of their assets, they cannot afford hospital-level care at all or are only be able to afford one period of hospitalization regardless of any need for further treatment. Insurance plans covering some of the costs of inpatient care are available for many Chinese urban dwellers, and there have been initial attempts to provide these in rural settings as well. This current situation, however, is inequitable, and it appears that Chinese health policies, as outlined in health reforms in 2009, and Malaysian health policies are designed to improve access to insurance products and decrease the cost of inpatient care for the rural poor.

PROFESSIONAL STANDARDS IN A CROSS-CULTURAL CONTEXT

The case studies from China, Cuba and India raise interesting questions about how to conduct an ethical analysis of law, policy and professional standards in cross-cultural contexts.

China

In China, basic ethical standards and practice regulations enacted in 1998 began to define and raise physician accountability. Physicians were not to exploit their position to extort money or suggest additional payments for services. However, as in many countries with a fee-for-service culture, physicians have financial incentives to: a) prescribe medications that require follow-up visits and repeat prescriptions, and b) perform additional procedures. Financial incentives to prescribe may be especially strong in China, as physicians sell medications from their own clinics. Because there is no government program to evaluate clinical and cost effectiveness, i.e. one comparable to that of NICE in the UK, there are reports in the media about physicians charging large fees for procedures that may be of dubious value to patients. Furthermore, and perhaps even worse, the practice of accepting "red envelopes" filled with money from grateful patients is still a widespread practice. Lastly, pharmaceutical corporation sponsorship of individual physician activities such as travel continue to be extended to physicians across China, whereas such practices are now banned in Britain and the US.

Although these actions would be deemed unethical in the West, are they unethical viewed from within in a Chinese context? Few of these actions might be found to directly contravene Chinese policy or protocol, leading one to ask what lens should be used for analyzing these activities. In other words, should Western standards apply, or should we be cautious in determining whether actions deemed as unethical in the West are deemed as unethical from within a Chinese cultural context?

As Chan suggests, under the Confucian ethical system, the most important ethical concern is whether the physician has acted with internal Confucian benevolence and professionalism, no matter what the economic impact of his or her actions. Using this virtue-ethics perspective, and in the absence of clear professional standards, it is not certain that such actions are indeed unethical in a Chinese context. Nonetheless, placed in the context of global standards, such as those adopted by the World Health Organization, the difference is marked, meaning that a decision has to made as to whether to adhere to universal, global standards, or to national, local standards. If so, it is not clear who would actually make that choice, or how such a decision would be implemented, especially if it meant widespread change to standards of practice.

This dichotomy applies to India as well as China, although in that instance standards have been set that are consistent with those set at the international level, it is just that they are frequently ignored. In moral terms, knowing that a system is in place and that standards exist but are not adhered to is perhaps worse than having no agreed standards; however, such analysis does not take account of the cultural dimensions of care provision and prevailing cultural values. The issue is therefore one of whether cultural context mitigates in some way the failure to adhere to international standards and protocols. The answer to this may well be no, even if there is clear evidence that cultural context influences how standards are framed and how they work in practice. At this level it is easier to make an assessment if one acknowledges local cultural influences and customs while evaluating professional practices.

In short, internationally agreed standards may be: a) accepted and adhered to; b) accepted but ignored; c) accepted and modified according to local custom, or d) totally ignored. Option a) may theoretically be the gold standard, but option c) is in some ways preferable, because here standards can be culturally sensitive and more relevant to specific population groups, focusing on the localized needs of patients. Option d) has little or nothing to bring to its defense, and option b) is especially challenging and points to significant problems with regulation and enforcement. Readers can by now probably place the countries studied here into the different categories.

Confucian values

The role of Confucian values in Chinese medical care includes many components of physician behavior that are similar to those in the West. The writings of Sun Simiao suggest that physicians should be competent, wise, sincere and demonstrate good will to their patients, and these are similar virtues to those contained within the Hippocratic Oath. While Western standards emphasize ethical behaviors in the context of the patient-physician relationship, Chinese standards prioritize the inner ethical duty of physicians to "comport themselves in a noble manner." This could have a real impact on how Chinese courts consider malpractice, whereby a physician may have thought his actions noble, yet adverse outcomes were nonetheless suffered by a patient. (In the West, motivations matter where criminal charges are being brought, otherwise patient outcomes tend to matter more, except where disciplinary charges are being brought—and in that case, it is physician insight that often makes the difference.)

Confucian standards may also influence the patient physician relationship. The high social standing of physicians and the power differential between them and their patients impact many aspects of this relationship. In the West, a dialogue between the physician and the patient is expected when developing a treatment plan that the patient endorses. In a traditional Confucian setting the physician would prescribe the treatment without any significant input from the patient. Furthermore, questions from the patient could be construed as questioning the integrity of the physician, who is expected to take everything into account and devise a benevolent treatment plan that the patient merely has to implement. A discussion of potential treatments and side effects, which is critical to informed consent in the West, would not be expected in a traditional Chinese ethical context. As Chan says, determining the ethical obligations of the physician in this context can be challenging.

The new criterion-based system for assessing physicians' professional behavior, included in the 2009 health reforms, covers traditional Confucian standards and Western-oriented standards, such as informed consent and confidentiality. These standards suggest that health policy leadership in China intends to implement a Western-oriented code of medical ethics. However, it is not yet clear whether the appearance of the words translated as "informed consent and confidentiality" in Chinese health policy mean that Chinese physicians will be expected to adhere to Western standards. Even if Chinese doctors are expected to do so, there will need to be a period for physician education about the ethical issues underlying informed consent and individual patient confidentiality. If these standards are implemented in China, further ethical analysis will be necessary to better understand how the current health care system can implement these standards. For example, how does one provide informed consent for treatment during an initial outpatient appointment lasting only five minutes? While the intention to implement these Western ethical standards may be noble, how they are interpreted and implemented will be critical to monitor.

Ethics in a time of war

In the Guantanamo case study, the United States government appears to posit that a different set of ethical principles can be applied because physicians and other medical staff at Guantanamo operate from within a different cultural context. The argument put forward suggests that in this context, i.e. the state of emergency following 9/11, usual laws, policies and professional standards do not pertain to Guantanamo Bay due to an extraordinary event that took place (namely, the 9/11 attacks on the United States). This cultural context argument was reinforced by staging interrogations in foreign countries, the argument being that if American physicians or medical staff were not physically in the United States, even if they were in the employ of the United States, then normal laws, policies and professional standards did not apply.

"Cultural context" in this case means something very different from what it can be taken to mean in other situations, where it is not being arbitrarily applied to people in military detention. Attempting to justify torture by these means makes a mockery of attempts to employ a culturally sensitive approach to the ethical analysis of health policy and professional standards, in that such actions significantly fail to withstand moral scrutiny of either Eastern or Western cultural origin. Therefore, in order for cultural context to be admissible within ethical discourse on standards of professionalism, it needs to be defined in ways that relate to how life is normally lived, not how normalcy is subverted in a time of war. A counter-argument could be that times of war always exist in some places and at some points in time; however, we do not believe that it is defensible to subvert international professional standards to the extent that performing acts that intentionally violate the human right of others can be ethically justified. To conclude otherwise is morally troubling and undermines the basic premise that culture makes a difference, for which some but not unlimited account should be taken.

India

The case study from India reinforces the importance of having a review process to clarify, prioritize and enforce complicated intersections of *personal* and *professional* ethical standards. These personal ethical standards may be based on personal religious beliefs regarded as being extremely important to particular individuals. In one example, drawn from the UK, a dentist was brought before the regulatory authority because he prioritized his own personal religious standards over his professional ethical obligations, refusing to treat women who did not wear traditional head covering in the form of culturally explicit clothing. The regulatory authority rightly determined that his professional obligations trumped his personal religious standards. Another case example, this time from India, offers a chance to review how terms like informed consent have different meanings in different cultural contexts. This case involved a young woman in labor and attempts to bring her to a birthing center where hi-tech, high-level interventions could be utilized. In this situation, significant delays occur because the woman is deemed unable to give informed consent solely by reason of her gender.

The rights of women in this setting are weak, and informed consent is often not possible for women on their own, especially if payment has to be authorized first. No treatment decision could be made without her husband, and his father too had to be consulted since he ultimately is paying for the care. The additional wait places the woman's life at risk, yet it appears that the physician is unable to intervene without first having "proper" authorization. In this case, the patient's rights are similar to those accorded to a child in many Western settings, whereby a young child is unable to make independent health care decisions. Since India is a signatory to World Health Organization and World Medical Council protocols, it is unlikely that this method of consent can be supported according to international professional standards. Rather, it is likely that the physician is responding to social pressure from the immediate family and the community in which the family lives. Since a) the doctor is a member of a nongovernmental organization [NGO] and thus not sponsored by government, and b) the physician, who is a foreign national, is giving her time, she is bound by her own professional standards and may be unfamiliar with local Indian ethical and legal frameworks. However, she judges that the operation of the NGO could be placed in jeopardy if she offends the community standard by seeking consent directly from the woman or by initiating action as an emergency. Women's rights are further discussed in the chapter on Malaysia, but in that case initiatives to improve access to services for women seem to be having good results, issues having more to do with unhealthy behaviors than with accessing basic services or the lack of personal autonomy.

It is possible that the Indian NGO depends on contributions from wealthy locals or from international donors who donate by reason of having religious or cultural affiliations. These donors may not be pleased if religious or cultural standards of the community are made subservient to national or international law, policy, professional standards or regulating authorities. Time-honored traditions are not easily displaced, and while no harm appears to have occurred because of the delay in this case, one wonders whether, in this extremely inaccessible part of India, had things gone wrong, what options would have been open to the family. Redress in the courts would have been difficult, partly because for this woman, she or her child could have died, and partly because the Indian court system is known for having long delays and so questions of access to the judicial system then arise.

THE LEGAL AND REGULATORY ENVIRONMENT

Chapter 2 reviewed intersections between ethics, policy and law as they exist in the West, noting how one function of society is to determine the standards and codes of conduct that pertain to health care. Mechanisms exist for adjudicating various aspects of policy and law, and we discussed jurisprudence on medical decision-making, as well as mechanisms for compensating individuals who have been harmed or otherwise disadvantaged by health policy and law, or by physician malpractice. This included setting standards for physicians communicating risk to a patient, and consultation practices for reviewing or even overturning ethical guidelines.

The dynamic relationship that exists between law and ethics may be viewed as integral to most Western views of civil society. However, institutions that establish law and policy and adjudicate on professional standards need to be robust. When these institutions do not function well, opportunities for remediation of damage done to an individual from not receiving care (or from receiving poor quality care) are limited, especially in a country such as India where the court system is not readily accessible and where medical regulation is weak.

Legal positivism is the preeminent (but not the only) legal philosophy in most modern liberal democracies. It provides a rationale for conceptions of morality at personal and state levels and how these impact on different members of society, including those involved in the organization and delivery of health care (even though this is not normally discussed in the literature on legal theory). Low levels of provision by the state and weak systems of justice can leave patients to fend for themselves, either through purchasing health care services directly or purchasing health care insurance. There is nothing wrong with either of these options as long as there is provision for those members of society least able to cope with accidental injury or ill-health. There are pitfalls too from having a centralized system of delivery that relies heavily on the state with inherently politicized control of health services.

Hierarchical, paternalistic decision-making impacts on the patient experience, and different approaches to patient autonomy can influence the course of events during a patient's journey through the various systems of health care provision. Too much individualized health care can come at the expense of the public interest, just as too much emphasis on public health and ready access can lead to poor quality care and less individual choice. Trying to enjoy the best of both approaches often implies a contradiction whereby policies that encourage one *discourage* the other; however, it is interesting to note that in emerging economies such as India and Malaysia, the tendency is increasingly towards a smaller role for the state sector in health provision. This trend may be inevitable and could well apply to other countries, but mechanisms must be in place in order to protect more vulnerable sectors in society.

In China, specific health policy and law may be either lacking or rarely enforced, and since so many changes have come about recently there is little precedent to guide health service providers and administrators. For example, there is no central and little provincial-level law or health policy directed towards care of the mentally ill. This means there is no consistent means for adjudicating difficult issues like involuntary commitment to a hospital for treatment, criminal responsibility while mentally ill, or the appointment of an individual to act in one's stead for financial or personal decision-making when mentally ill.

Professional standards for physicians have been relatively recently enacted in China, and while strong central governmental control means that promulgation of the standards is likely to be widespread, enforcement may be weakened by the tendency not to criticize the behavior of another professional. These attitudes may be rooted in memories of the denunciation of professionals during the Cultural Revolution, or rooted in traditions that tend to revere elders, and so they may feature strongly in people's minds.

In India, professional standards are consistent with those standards set by bodies such as the international organizations. However, as already seen, individual Indian physicians may not be well educated on these codes of conduct; instead they often have an individualistic sense of standard-setting, which can weaken the implementation of these standards. Reported ethical problems within the Medical Council of India, the institution that regulates medical care in India, further exacerbate these problems. In contrast to China, where the central government sets policy and law, in India much of the power for setting, interpreting and enforcing law, policy and standards is reserved for the States, furthering the potential for standards to be either not set clearly or enforced.

Moreover, India and China both acknowledge difficulties with their citizens having access to the legal system, especially for those living in the countryside. Where written law or policy does exist there is no guarantee that an individual will be able to access the legal system (although improvements in access are being made in both countries). In China, there has been a tradition of travelling to Beijing to seek redress on policy issues or administrative rulings that have negatively affected individuals, but this petitioner system of seeking justice is increasingly being discouraged. However, Chinese health reforms enacted in 2009 include measures to improve the transparency of complaints procedures, which should help improve access to institutions that can adjudicate on health care difficulties. In both China and India, improved access to adjudication systems is critical to mitigating risk and seeking redress for those harmed by health law, policy or negligent medical practice.

The Guantanamo case study makes it clear that difficulty with the legal and regulatory environment is not solely a problem for the developing world. This serves as an important reminder that ethical analyses, using law, policy and professional standards as a guide, need to ensure that the process of developing law, policy and standards is, in and of itself, fair and consistent with other established ethical standards and norms. There were significant problems in the process of upholding standards when they are applied in Guantanamo in such a way as to distort the original intention of standards and regulatory mechanisms.

These policy and standards changes were developed in secret, allegedly under pressure from the highest levels of the Bush administration. The policies and standards flouted US-approved international doctrines on the ethical treatment of prisoners and the protection of human rights. These changes were made under the pretext that the Taliban had contravened the Geneva Convention first, which provided dubious precedent for the US to act in the way it did. The dissemination of changes to indoctrination manuals were communicated to the field, while the official public stance remained that torture was not allowed. Attempts to obtain information about the nature of the interrogations were consistently resisted on the basis of national security concerns. Only later when the public outcry intensified and when there was an election on the horizon, was clear repudiation of these policies actually accomplished.

CONFLICTS OF INTEREST IN THE DOCTOR-PATIENT RELATIONSHIP

The case studies from the United States cause us to pay attention to the importance of ethical analysis as part of the whole process of health policy development. They raise questions about how significant conflicts of interest can exist in a country where medical practice is highly regulated and where clear codes of professional behavior exist. The Guantanamo case study convincingly rejects the idea that "dual loyalty" obligations to both a patient and a third party, or to a patient and a broader social purpose, as exemplified by the requirement to report child abuse, can justify the abrogation of ethical duties, allowing torture to be carried out for the purposes of national security. Military physicians, who have been shown to be bound by the same ethical obligations as civilian physicians, are sworn to uphold the Constitution, which prohibits torture, and they must be able to recognize when a dual loyalty argument contravenes longstanding, agreed professional standards.

Chapters by Hussain and Broughton reinforce the importance of disclosing and understanding potential conflicts of interest and methods for the management of such conflicts when conducting policy analysis. The effect of conflicts of interest on the iron triangle, the effectiveness of appeals to the judiciary in mitigating the effect of these ethical lapses, and extending the lessons learned in the US to other countries are all important elements to consider.

Hussain documents the ethical challenges facing physicians who participate in clinical research sponsored by pharmaceutical companies. Conflicts of interest occur when physicians are paid to do research at the same time as providing clinical care for patients—the same patients who are participating in trials. Practices like compensating physicians for the recruitment of subjects into research protocols place the physician's financial interests at odds with the best interests of their patients. The relationship patients have with their physicians makes the consent process particularly challenging when it is difficult for physicians to encourage trial participation without limiting patient rights to autonomy.

Codes of conduct governing both the corporation and the physician exist at many levels (including federal and state regulations, and voluntary codes of conduct governing both corporations and physicians). Universities have also attempted to manage these ethical conflicts by requiring academic physicians to disclose their financial relationships with industry. However, as Hussain documents, enforcement of these codes and policies has been lax at all levels, and as recent disclosures of impropriety have demonstrated, many of those involved in research have financial interests with pharmaceutical corporations.

Broughton documents similar ethical concerns about bias resulting from the financial relationship between the pharmaceutical industry and the provision of continuing medical education for physicians in the US. Again, voluntary codes of conduct exist at corporate level, at the education accreditation agency, and at university level, and the physician groups like the American Medical Association regulate this kind of activity. However, reports of physicians receiving large consulting and speaking fees from industry, as well as documented evidence of physicians receiving these fees favoring prescription of high-cost drugs or use of medical devices favored by industry, have provoked public outcry. It is now generally accepted that these voluntary codes have been ineffective in fully controlling both corporate and individual physician behavior.

What is the effect of these conflicts of interest on access, quality and cost of care? It seems likely that quality and cost are most influenced. The conflicts of interest between industry and individual physicians and their patients suggest that medical research financed by corporations is biased in favor of finding positive outcomes for new drugs or medical devices. This risks negatively impacting quality of care by introducing new products which are not clearly superior to existing products, and since new products often cost more to purchase due to patent laws in the US, this bias has very significant cost effects.

Would an ethical analysis of the policies governing the relationship between pharmaceutical corporations and physicians conducting research or continuing medical education have predicted these conflicts?

Might regulations to mitigate the effect of these conflicts have prevented the raft of negative publicity which has damaged public trust in the medical research endeavor and trust that advice from physicians is unbiased by payment from outside agencies?

These questions arise during a time when regulation of many economic relationships and practices is being rethought. The home mortgage crisis and the subsequent collapse of the financial industry and the broader economy have many similarities to conflicts of interest between individual physician behavior and corporate profits in the medical profession and pharmaceutical industry. In both instances corporations provided incentives that encouraged behavior that undermined fiduciary duties. As re-regulation of the financial industry derives more support, perhaps this resolve will be generalized to develop increased regulation of the relationship between physicians and pharmaceutical corporations. Recent experience suggests that regulation and enforcement may need to improve simultaneously in order to have an effect on behavior.

When bias in medical research can be established as a policy consciously propagated by industry, states in the US (that pay for the improperly approved medications or devices through Medicaid health insurance entitlements for the indigent) may seek redress through the courts. This causes one to ask what role the legal system plays in redressing these ethical breeches. There have been reports that states' attorney generals are considering such action to recoup costs, and if successful, it is likely that these actions will spur corporations to deal more aggressively with biases in research. While some academics have had to resign from their university positions due to failing to disclose the extent of their relationships with industry, we are not aware of pending lawsuits against them personally over their actions.

If the legal system has been ineffective in spurring reform, what initiatives have been suggested and what has motivated the changes?

Various methods have been suggested to improve oversight and mitigate the effect of these ethical conflicts of interest. Corporations have attempted to manage them by contracting with independent agencies to sponsor clinical trials. Attempts to mitigate publication biases require authors to disclose their financial relationships with corporations sponsoring their study at the time of publication, and to not lend their name to ghostwritten manuscripts. Notification of post-approval drug side effects may be improved by mandating post-approval studies of the medication. Development of policies concerning industry contributions to continuing medical education attempt to dissociate contributions to education from practices that are clearly in the interests of corporations. Many interventions have been devised following unfavorable publicity, for example, those spurred by the 2008–2009 Congressional committee hearings.

How might the lessons learned from experiences in the US be transferred to medical systems in other countries?

Marienfeld reports conflicts between pharmaceutical industry and physicians in China similar to those outlined by Hussein and Broughton in the US. Interestingly, it would appear that the self-regulation that corporations have imposed on their US operations do not apply to international operations in China. The Chinese health reforms of 2009 appear to recognize the problem, providing evidence of a determination to eliminate reimbursement schemes provided by pharmaceutical companies to physicians and hospitals. Corporations should surely use the same ethical standards in international settings that they use in the US and UK.

Prospective, progressive regulation may be able to protect patient interests and prevent levels of public distrust in China and the rest of the developing world that have clouded medical practice and research in the US. Recent reports of attacks on doctors by patients and their family members underscore the fragile nature of the doctor-patient relationship in China. Whether and by what mechanism these regulations will be enforced is therefore as much of an issue in the developing world as it is in the US. Federal levels of regulation may be less likely in a decentralized country such as India and in other countries in the developing world. As pharmaceutical companies move research and drug development to the developing world (ostensibly for cost reasons), developing methods to regulate and enforce ethical conduct of research and clinical practice in these countries is something that has become urgent.

While overt pharmaceutical sponsorship of research and continuing medical education programs has been the focus to date when conducting an ethical analysis, the possibility of other covert conflicts of interest needs investigating. The growth of independent companies contracted by the pharmaceutical corporations to conduct their studies or manage their relationships with continuing medical education is one such potential covert source of conflict.

Furthermore, one should look carefully at the financing of NGOs, which have assumed roles in providing care and conducting research. The ARROW program in Malaysia discloses its funders on its website, much like the transparency that is being sought in ensuring physicians disclose their relationships with pharmaceutical corporations in continuing medical education and research publication settings. It is our view that the transparency at ARROW provides a model that other NGOs should seek to emulate.

INTEGRATING PUBLIC OPINION INTO RISK ASSESSMENT STRATEGIES

Lee and Marfeo review risk assessment policies and procedures in two developed countries: Italy and the UK. Marfeo documents the scientific literature on electroconvulsive therapy (ECT) for depression, finding it to be quite effective and producing fewer side effects in certain patient populations. Despite these scientific findings of effectiveness, the National Bioethics Committee of Italy ruled that ECT should be used with caution to assure the "safeguarding of a patient's personality and dignity." ECT was to be utilized only with supervision and consultation from local ethics committees. It seems likely that negative public perceptions of ECT, reinforced by media depictions of the procedure and widely held beliefs that psychiatric illness is caused by social problems that can be solved through social struggle and revival of the patient's aggressiveness influenced this decision in Italy. Unfortunately, while the care of patients with mental disorders is a required health benefit in Italy, the provision of ECT is not; these ethical recommendations to seek consultation may become barriers to a more patient-oriented discussion of safe, effective treatments for depression.

Lee finds similar outcomes in the UK, where NICE and the various regulatory bodies tend to adopt formulaic, top-down approaches to risk, typically intended to minimize negative outcomes. These risk-averse, blanket regulations place pressure on physicians to meet performance-based goals, which can undermine incentives to engage in more individualized approaches to risk, i.e. ones that are patient-centered.

Comparisons of this top-down, highly regulated approach to managing risk are quite different from approaches taken in China, where Traditional Chinese Medicine (TCM) is integrated with allopathic Western-style medicine. Interventions utilized in TCM have by and large not been tested by standard, randomized, controlled trial methodologies, and so effectiveness and risk are often not well delineated, when viewed from a science perspective. However, from a public opinion perspective, the belief that these treatments have been successfully used over hundreds of years leads individuals into also believing in the effectiveness of treatment, often explicitly requesting TCM interventions.

Chinese physicians manage this dilemma by prescribing allopathic treatment and helping the patient to access TCM interventions as complementary treatment, making referrals to a TCM provider as required. In Chinese medical schools and academic centers, there are departments of TCM where therapeutic values of these interventions are being evaluated. In this instance, lack of centralized, top-down law, policy and standards is a benefit, affording physicians the freedom to utilize more patient-oriented approaches towards the assessment of risk.

While this freedom to incorporate individual patient beliefs into the treatment plan offers certain advantages, the tradition of TCM is not without its own ethical dilemmas. For example, the TCM physician is expected to prescribe a treatment for patients during their visit; this tradition continues to play out in patient expectations of the role of the physician as always prescribing some sort physical remedy.

This set of patient expectations about the role of the physician places the Chinese physician in an ethical dilemma, as patients may feel that their physician is not "a good doctor" if they are asked to leave without a prescription. Additionally, the tradition that *more* expensive interventions are better than *less* expensive interventions is also problematic, as patients feel less invested in the process when they receive the more cost-effective medical intervention, challenging common perceptions that expensive medicines are invariably "best." Many TCM interventions have not been studied or proven to be clinically effective, and as China moves toward a more Western-oriented model of allopathic health care and develops more health care-related law and policy, it will be interesting to monitor how TCM is viewed in the future, and how much it will be integrated into care for each individual patient.

SUMMARY

The intent of this book is to demonstrate the utility of using health care law, policy and professional standards as a means to effect practical analysis of the ethical issues that arise in the provision of health services. Rather than relying on moral absolutes, we believe that examination of health law, policy and professional standards offers an opportunity to view how society decides to codify beliefs in a way that is pertinent to ethical analysis. Since law, policy and professional standards have to deal with real-life issues, ethical analysis that is based on these frameworks may offer more practical solutions than one based on moral absolutes, and it can be more sensitive to the nuances of culture in different settings (provided of course that they have not been subverted to accord with immoral means and ends, as evidenced at Guantanamo).

Overall, we believe this methodology for analysis is supported by the findings of the case studies, and analysis of these case studies suggests five questions, which should be carefully considered when conducting ethical analysis in this way:

1   Were laws, policies and professional standards developed in a transparent manner with input from necessary stakeholders, suggesting that the frameworks adopted offer a fair representation of societal values (remembering to check

whether they are consistent with other ethical frameworks to which that society is a signatory)?

2   Are ethical frameworks that have been adopted by society able to respond to rapid change when this occurs, and are other historical frameworks pertinent or viewed as being predominant in society? How might they be employed?

3   As new law, policies and standards are deployed, how are clinicians and administrators educated about new standards? When Western-oriented terms are utilized in the standard, what do those terms mean in practice? Does the health care practice model support the intention of the new law, policy or standards or is it highly unlikely that new policies can be successfully implemented?

4   Are other interested parties unduly influencing the development of law, policy, professional standards, or processes of implementation and regulatory review? Are there any overt or covert conflicts of interest present, and how are conflicts of interest managed when they do present? By the same token, those responsible for doing ethical analysis should disclose their conflicts of interest, such as sources of support for the author in question or for agencies that the author represents.

5   Are there mechanisms that enable one to appeal to regulatory authorities to help clarify the intent of a policy and mitigate any harms that come about through policies being in force? What remedies are proposed by relevant regulatory authorities?

Having in mind these questions may prove to be of practical use to policy analysts and policy decision-makers in the future, thus enabling them to help plan interventions and meet patients' needs more effectively.

ENDNOTES

1   The authors would like to thank Deans and Heads of School at Yale and Keele University Schools of Medicine for support in helping us establish and run the medical student exchange program and in terms of our respective programs of research, enabling us to write the book.

2   The authors are grateful to each of the contributors. In addition, they would like to thank Dr Sonia Chery for kindly providing case examples and important background information for the chapter on India.

3   The authors hope that this book will prove useful to readers as they consider these various ethical issues, which are at the intersection of health law, policy and professional practice. They would be pleased to hear from readers who wish to share their experiences on the topics raised in this book.

Index